
- Fines for late returns are charged per item, per day.

- Two week loan items can be renewed if they have not been requested by another borrower **www.staffs.ac.uk/borrowing**

- One day and two day loan items cannot be renewed and must be returned to the site where they were issued.

M8178

Chronic Pain Management:
The Essentials

Paul AJ Hardy
BSc(HONS), MB, CHB, MD, MA, FRCA

Consultant in Pain Management
Gloucestershire Royal Hospital, Gloucester, UK

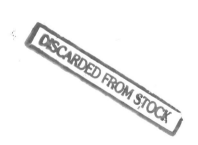

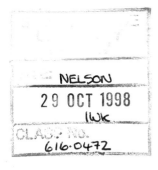

© 1997

Greenwich Medical Media

507 The Linen Hall

162-168 Regent Street

London

W1R 5TB

ISBN 1 900 151 855

First Published 1997

Distributed worldwide by

Oxford University Press

Production and Design

Derek Virtue, DataNet

Printed in Great Britain by

Ashford Colour Press Limited

Contents

Basic Concepts

What is Pain?

This fundamental question has challenged philosophers over the centuries. Of all the sensations it is one where there is not a just adequate stimulus, for example pain does not equal a factor x, such that removal of x produces relief of pain. It is a sensation where other inputs such as emotional distress or spiritual distress may invoke the same overall feeling as a physical injury.

An individuals pain response may also vary in time. The response may appear inconsistent, for example how can someone claim to be in pain yet laugh or smile? It is clear that this feeling is not just a physical sensation, or an emotion or a psychological disturbance but a combination of all of these. Not only is pain a complex function of physical, emotional and psychological factors but it is internal, it cannot be measured or demonstrated externally.

The concept about pain is important because it leads on to how to approach a patient and how to deal with for example chronic pain. In these patients not only may there not be an obvious reason for the complaint but there is in most cases not an 'analgesic' treatment. The greatest danger for both the physician and the patient is to deal with the chronic pain patient as if they had acute pain. This results in unnecessary and futile treatments and may encourage the patients abnormal behaviour perpetuating their particular problem.

Anatomy of Pain

The classical anatomical pathway of nociception involves the excitation of certain peripheral axons. There is not a defined

Fibre Type	Diameter (μ)	Myelination	Conduction velocity (m/sec)	Function
Aα	6-22	+	30-120	motor, proprioception
Aβ	6-22	+	30-120	motor, proprioception
Aγ	3-6	+	15-35	muscle spindle afferents
Aδ	1-4	+	5-25	sensory afferents
B	<3	+	3-15	preganglionic sympathetic
C	0.3-1.3	–	0.7-1.3	sensory afferent
C	0.4-1.2	–	0.1-2.0	postganglionic sympathetic

Table 1 – Nerve fibre types

nociceptor. There are several different nerve fibre types with differing diameter, myelination and conduction velocity (Table 1). This is apparent as a 'fast' pain component which is thought to be via larger myelinated fibres and a 'slow' pain component which is thought to be via small unmyelinated fibres.

The incoming nerve fibres enter and synapse in the posterior horn of the spinal cord where there is a 'gating' or switch mechanism. The relative balance of incoming information at this level determines whether a pain signal is transmitted higher into the central nervous system.

The classical nociceptor pathway involves crossing over of the secondary neuron within the spinal cord at some point over 5-7 spinal segments to ascend in the contralateral anterolateral white matter of the cord. There is a semi somatotopic representation of the body within the spinothalamic tract which may be interrupted during cordotomy procedures. The spinothalamic tract terminates within the thalamic nuclei and third order neurons project from there onto the sensory cortex.

The thalamus is at the junction of the sensory systems and the limbic system which is involved in emotion. It is therefore of no surprise that there is an interrelationship between pain and emotion.

Recent interest has concentrated on some of the further linkages in this system and in particular the involvement of descending control mechanisms. These arise through lateral branching of the primary and secondary sensory neurons which transmit both ipsilateral and contralateral information to other thalamic and brainstem nuclei from which descending tracts originate. These mechanisms have been well studied in animals in which they explain most if not all of the basis behind electrical stimulation methods. In addition to the discrete descending pathways there are diffuse inhibitory control pathways which may be recruited with a sufficient stimulus.

A further area of interest has arisen out of the need to explain certain phenomena of chronic pain and its treatment. Interest has centered around the spinal cord layers involved in the pain transmission and recognition that the secondary neurons respond to a wide range of stimuli, that is they are not just nociceptive. The balance of inputs onto these 'wide dynamic range' neurons determines onward transmission.

Despite advances in imaging technology we are no further to resolving where in the brain pain is perceived and processed. There is involvement of the thalamic nuclei, the limbic system, the periaqueductal gray and the sensory and frontal cortex.

Physiology of Pain

There are several physiological principles involved in nociception. Neuronal transmission may be varied by the number of inputs and collateral branching of axons which allow for amplification and deamplification of the incoming information. The system is not hard wired, therefore recurrent information may lead to the development of preferential nerve pathways or atrophy of the alternative routes. Stimulation of smaller circuits may lead to augmentation of the input which has been implicated in the development of wind-up, with persistent neuronal loops. These have not been demonstrated anatomically but are hypothesized from the physiological experiments and have been proposed to explain persistent pain and the neurogenic phenomena of allodynia and hyperpathia.

The lack of hard-wiring also allows for the concept of neuroplasticity. This is the proposed mechanism whereby the central nervous system responds to a constant presence of or lack of stimulus. It has been shown that secondary neurons may respond to a variable peripheral field over time. It has also been shown that after amputation of digits that the part of the nervous system which used to respond to that body part starts to respond to alternative stimuli, which may be far removed from the original. For example a somatic area, in for example the thalamus, may start to respond to a visceral stimulus. This plasticity may account for return of pain after certain lesions or treatments and some of the strange phenomena which have been reported, for example mirror image pain after cordotomy.

Another field of interest, particularly in relation to visceral and joint pain, is the concept of silent nociceptors. There are many nerve axons within the tissues which when tested do not have any resting neural activity. Under certain circumstances, for example ischaemia, activity may be detected. It is thought that these silent nociceptors remain inactive until there is a sufficient combination of stimuli and humeral factors to activate the nociceptor.

Pharmacology

The neurophysiology and pharmacology of pain are inter-twined. Investigations over the last decades have shown that there are transmitter 'soups' both peripherally and centrally rather than discrete pharmacologic targets.

Peripherally there are a series of tissue factors — autacoids and leukotrines - which may be released in tissues during experimental studies. Some of these may be usefully inhibited or blocked, such as the prostaglandins, whereas others have other effects which inhibit targeting of them or where known inhibitors do not exist. Interestingly some agents which were thought to be purely central, such as opioids, have been shown to have clinically useful peripheral activity.

In the central nervous system far more has been learnt about for example the various drug actions on the spinal cord but there is also much which is yet unknown. Known transmitter chemicals involved in nociceptive pathways include opioids, adrenergic, cholinergic, glutaminergic, glycine and neuropep-tides such as substance P, somatostatin and calcitonin. The prostaglandins which were for a long time assumed to be peripherally acting are now know to also have direct central effects.

Within the system there are checks and balances. Alpha-adrenergic drugs are analgesic in the spinal cord but nocigenic at higher centres. The balance of agents may be important for example opioids may stimulate both 'off-cells' to provide analgesia and 'on-cells' to enhance nociception.

The concept of neuroplasticity has been enhanced by the findings that opioids, glutamate and substance P are all contained within the C-fibres entering the spinal cord. The glutamate receptor (NMDA) is present on the C-fibre membrane (pre-synaptic). The neuron therefore stimulates itself to release further transmitter. Substance P is present in the axons of the C-fibres, within the substantia gelatinosa of the spinal cord, yet the receptors for this transmitter are present over the axonal surface of deeper layer neurons. There is no simple synapse with this transmitter but rather a diffusion within the spinal cord. Chronic pretreatment with opioid leads to enhanced sensitivity to substance P ipsi- and contralaterally within the cord.

Recent research has led to an increased understanding of some mechanisms of nociception, particularly in animal preparations, but have not led to any significant new therapies.

Measurement of Pain

Pain is not just a sensation and there are no external markers suitable for measurement. In the awake adult the presence of pain is relatively easy to assess but in the unconscious, the very young or the otherwise incompetent patient in whom simple communication is difficult then it may be imperative to rely on changes in physiological functions. Pain may produce reflex autonomic changes such as increases in heart rate or blood pressure, increased respiratory rate or dilation of the pupils and sweating. The problem with these changes is that they may also occur for reasons other than pain per se. For example these changes may occur in the otherwise adequately anaesthetised patient.

Pain scales have been developed to put a numerical score on the perception. The simplest system is to ask for the presence or absence of pain. An extension of this is to breakdown the presence on a simple verbal rating, for example none, mild, moderate, severe and excruciating. These systems can cause problems if the patient and rater have different concepts of the words used – is mild less than or greater than moderate?

An extension of the rating scale is the visual analogue scale. These are used in a variety of guises including lines marked from 0-100 mm to happy through sad faces and colour scaling systems. There is an assumption in the use of such scales that they are linear scales, although most sensory functions are actually exponential mathematically.

An inverse visual analogue is the pain relief score where decrements of pain are measured rather than degree of pain present. These may be combined over time to assess "area under the curve" of pain presence or of analgesia. These make assumptions about the change of pain over time as well as the assumed linearity of the sensation.

These tools are ideally suited to assessing pain in the acute setting. They are totally inadequate in the chronic pain patient as they fail to address the multidimensional nature of the pain response in these patients. In addition they tend to concentrate on introspection by the patient on the pain complaint and are potentially harmful for these patients.

More complex pain scoring systems have included the multifactorial 'McGill pain questionnaire' this uses multiple descriptive words ranked into subgroups by type of description, and grouped together under sensory, evaluative and affective descriptors. although cumbersome this provides more useful information about individual pain problems. This has advantages in chronic pain where pain patterns may be recognised. Furthermore the McGill questionnaire has been translated into several languages allowing cross cultural reference and study.

Improvements in assessment can be obtained by including a function of activity and measure of pain relieving factors. Activity rating scales are important in the conscious as well as in those with reduced autonomy. Pain during coughing, whilst walking, etc. or measured by way of force of expiration (Peak flow) or walking distances give valuable additional information. Consumption of analgesic over time gives further information about particular pain problems although there are great inter-individual variations.

pain — Depression

Psychological function is affected by pain and pain is affected by psychological function. A variety of scoring systems have been developed to assess for example anxiety, or depression. These are particularly valuable in chronic pain complaints where the degree of suffering may be modified by treatment but the pain score remains the same. There are simple systems, for example the Hospital Anxiety and Depression scale, and more complex tools for example the Hamilton Depression scale. Other tools which may have a role include quality of life, Pain Disability Index, Sickness Impact Profiles and Locus of Control measures (Table 2).

Pain intensity	Numerical rating scales
	Visual analogue scales
	Verbal rating scales
	Pain drawings
	McGill questionnaire
Functional Capacity	Sickness impact profile
	Short-form health surveys
	Multidimensional inventory
	Pain disability index
Mood and personality	Minnesota multiphasic inventory (MMPI)
	Beck depression inventory
	Strait-trait anxiety inventory
	Illness behaviour questionnaire
	Symptom checklist 90
	Hospital anxiety and depression scale
Pain beliefs and coping	Coping strategies questionnaires
	Pain management inventory
	Pain self-efficacy questionnaire
	Pain attitudes survey
	Negative thoughts inventory
Medication	Medication record
Psychosocial	Comprehensive pain questionnaire

Table 2 – Assessment categories and scales

Although more commonly used in chronic and cancer pain settings these psychological tools are of great value in the acute pain setting, for example anxiety level may influence the use of patient controlled analgesic consumption. Locus of control has an effect on the success of postoperative pain control method.

Acute Pain

Types of Pain

There are two fundamental types of pain and four subtypes of each of these. There is an extra subgrouping based upon response to treatment. This differentiation is of practical importance because of the methods of pain management which follow on from the typing of the pain. Of course there are occasions in which there is more than one type of pain present. Individual patients do not neatly occupy particular niches, however the individual contributing pains can be individually treated to allow a more holistic approach.

The two main types of pain are those of ACUTE and CHRONIC pain. These are the types of pain not a measure of the degree of pain. There are four further subtypes of pain – NOCIGENIC, BEHAVIOURAL, NEUROGENIC and PSYCHOGENIC. The separate subgrouping is of PARADOXICAL pains.

Acute pain is pain which occurs at the time of and immediately after a particular injury or disease process – for example chest pain with myocardial infarction or limb pain after a fracture. This type of pain may persist through the healing phase of the disease process, that is during the first 2-3 months. In some conditions acute pain may persist or be recurring, for example joint pain in arthritis which recurs every time the joint is moved. Persistent acute pain includes ischaemic pain and cancer pain. Analgesia, that is the complete removal of pain may be possible in acute pain conditions. Preventative treatments may be possible, before the pain process, for example the use of local anaesthetic creams before venepuncture.

Acute pain is associated with the release of peripheral and central chemical mediators the object of which is to encourage inactivity of the person to allow healing and recovery from disease. The chemicals released by the nervous system may also induce analgesia in themselves and may induce changes in mood which encourage immobility.

Chronic pain in contrast to this is pain which persists beyond the usual healing phase of the disease process. The change to chronicity is accompanied by changes in mobility, encouraging rest when activity should be resumed. There may be major psychological impairment with the use of abnormal behaviours and thoughts. The immobility produces effects on mood and

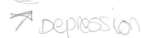

induces physiological changes which reinforce the persistence of pain. Chronic pain is characterised by patient distress rather than pain. Many of the changes which take place in chronic pain can be identified in patients with persistent acute or recurrent acute pain complaints and in cancer pain.

Nocigenic pain is pain associated with stimulation of the classical pain pathways from the peripheral receptor. Most pains associated with injury and disease are nocigenic, at least in the initial stages. This type of pain can be treated using methods directed at the classical pain pathway notably pain killers and nerve blocks. With the development of chronicity these methods generally become ineffective.

Behavioural pain starts as nocigenic pain which is then associated with changes in behaviour, which in themselves may be overt or covert. Overt behaviours are those in which an external behaviour is associated with pain and in which avoidance of the behaviour may reduce the pain problem. A full assessment is essential since in some cases the patient needs to persist with the activity and find other methods of reducing the pain intensity. Covert behaviour is typified by 'illness behaviours' which are patterns of behaviour which appear to be changed due to the pain although there is no anatomical or physiological basis for the change. Conventional analgesics and nerve blocks are positively dangerous in these pain conditions since they reinforce the abnormal responses of the patient and prevent adequate rehabilitation. Psychological and stimulation techniques are the mainstay of therapy.

Neurogenic pain is pain occurring as a consequence of damage to the nervous system, either peripherally or centrally. Damage to he peripheral nervous system is associated initially with some nocigenic components but typically progresses over an interval of 3-6 months to lose these attributes and become purely neurogenic. In this type of pain there is usually associated sensory disturbances and may be motor and autonomic disturbance. Various sensory abnormalities occur ranging from anaesthesia, or absence of sensation, to hyperaesthesia, or increased sensation. Paraesthesia, or changed sensation, may occur spontaneously or after a stimulus and if it is unpleasant it is known as dysaesthesia. Allodynia is when a normally non-painful stimulus is perceived as pain, hyperpathia is when

use this as mindful example maybe.

there is an increased duration and intensity to a perceived sensation despite a brief stimulus. There must be evidence of some structural damage to the peripheral or central nervous system. As it may be predicted from a process which arises from damage to the pain pathways this type of pain does not respond to classical analgesics. There may be a response to centrally acting drugs. Some types of central pain respond to physical treatments.

Psychogenic pain is that pain which occurs as a form of mental illness or process. It may be associated with psychosis, for example the pain may be delusional, or with hysterical illness. This category should not be used as a medical 'dustbin' but should be based upon full psychiatric assessment.

Paradoxical pain may be from any of the foregoing categories but has the paradox that it may be made worse by an analgesic and need treating by an antalgesic. This type of pain may develop due to interference by metabolites of the active analgesic or may have been paradoxical all along. Specialist help may be required to diagnose and treat the patient.

Pain Treatments

There are several approaches used which each have their own end points. Analgesia, or the removal of pain, may be possible with acute pain. "Pain relief" is a reduction of the pain level not the removal of pain. "Pain management" is concerned with the reduction of suffering and enhanced quality of life rather than a reduction in the pain complaint. Pain management is central to the treatment of chronic, that is long duration, pain.

Several aspects of the pain treatment are important but are frequently overlooked. Many factors are involved in medical treatment which are not specific. Reduction in pain due to a non-specific action of the treatment, the placebo action is common and may occur in up to 100% of cases treated. There is no simple method to screen out this effect which may arise due to a variety of mechanisms. If the treatment itself is noxious, as for example surgery or injections, then a similar effect, known as a nocebo, may occur. For many of the methods described in this book the result of the "treatment" may be a consequence of either of these effects. As more techniques are investigated in depth these non-specific factors start to dominate the results. Epidural injections for back pain and sympathetic blocks for so-called sympathetic mediated pain (defined by the response to an uncontrolled injection) are examples where these non-specific actions may be the predominant action.

Other nonspecific actions may occur with a particular treatment, for example any substance injected into the body may act through systemic absorption rather than by a direct pharmacological or physical method. It is important to try and define which aspect of a treatment is actually effective in an attempt to gain benefits with decreased risks to the patient.

Management of Pain Types

Acute Pain

Acute pain lasting hours to days may be better prevented with preemptive analgesia. Procedural pain may be prevented with local blocks and treated with short acting agents such as alfentanyl, ketamine and nitrous oxide. For pain lasting hours to days use the appropriate level of the analgesic staircase. Continuous delivery using sustained release preparations or infusions are better.

With local anaesthetic techniques infusion into plexuses or spinal canal may provide better continuous control. Adequate volume of solution of the adequate concentration is required at the right level, for example thoracic epidural analgesia for thoracic incisions.

Analgesic Summary:

Analgesics	Simple	
	NSAIDs	Chapter 3
	Opioids including PCA and continuous infusions	
	Inhalational	
Physical	Local Anaesthetic Blocks	Chapter 5
	Spinal drug delivery	
		Chapter 4
	Stimulation Techniques TENS, Acupuncture	

Chronic Pain

a) Nocigenic Pain

In nocigenic pain there is stimulation of peripheral receptors, conduction of axonal traffic along peripheral nerves to the spinal cord with gated entry and onward transmission to higher centres. Much is known about the neurotransmitters involved and of the anatomical nerve pathways. In certain cases, for example in cardiac ischaemic pain, treatment of the underlying medical condition will reduce pain. In other cases management of pain is by analgesic drugs, nerve blocking and stimulation techniques.

A few do's and do not's. If using opioids do give an effective dose with effective dose increments. Do not give subcutaneous infusions or fentanyl patches simply because the patient has a diagnosis of cancer – oral morphine is well tolerated and should be used while the patient can take oral medication. Do not mix opioids particularly with reference to breakthrough medication – give the patient a small dose of the maintenance drug to take. Do not use mixed agonist antagonist or partial agonist drugs – they have no advantages over the straight agonists.

With NSAIDs use one at a time – mixing agents confers no advantages and may speed the onset of problems. Remember NSAIDs are not muscle relaxants. Also remember creams are absorbed and all forms may affect the gastrointestinal tract – you do not have to take the drug orally to get ulcers!

Analgesic Summary:

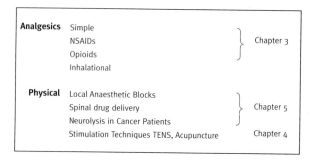

Analgesics	Simple	
	NSAIDs	} Chapter 3
	Opioids	
	Inhalational	
Physical	Local Anaesthetic Blocks	
	Spinal drug delivery	} Chapter 5
	Neurolysis in Cancer Patients	
	Stimulation Techniques TENS, Acupuncture	Chapter 4

CHRONIC RECURRENT NOCIGENIC PAIN

Analgesics	Simple	Chapter 3
	NSAIDs	
Physical	Stimulation Analgesia TENS, Acupuncture, SCS	Chapter 4
	Local Anaesthetic Blocks	Chapter 5

Examples:

CANCER PAIN

pharmacology	analgesic staircase. There is no maximum dose for opioids.	Chapter 3
	Give appropriate doses regularly to avoid breakthrough pain.	
	antidepressants, anticonvulsants for nerve pain	
	steroids for nerve and visceral pain and raised intracranial pressure	
	hormonal therapy and chemotherapy for appropriate pain	
physical	radiotherapy	
	stimulation – TENS, acupuncture	Chapter 4
	spinal drug delivery	Chapter 5
	nerve blockade for mechanical, visceral, nerve infiltration	
	cordotomy for unilateral body pain	
psychology	screening and support as required	

PERIPHERAL VASCULAR PAIN

pharmacology	analgesic staircase	Chapter 3
	vasodilators	
	anticoagulation as required	
physical	surgical repair, revascularisation and amputation as required	
	sympathectomy	Chapter 5
	stimulation – SCS, TENS	Chapter 4
physical therapy	as indicated	

CARDIAC ISCHAEMIC PAIN

pharmacology	analgesic staircase	Chapter 3
	cardiac vasodilators	
physical	surgical revasularisation as required	
	stimulation – SCS, TENS	Chapter 4
psychology	stress management	Chapter 6
	rehabilitation	
physical therapy	rehabilitation programme	Chapter 6,7

ARTHRITIS

pharmacology	simple analgesic, NSAIDs	
	antidepressants	Chapter 3
physical	splints and braces	Chapter 7
	orthopaedic assessment	
	nerve blocks for acute crises and	
	inoperable cases	Chapter 5
physical therapy	as appropriate	

CRANIOFACIAL PAIN

pharmacology	simple analgesics	
	antidepressants	Chapter 3
	anticonvulsants	
physical	maxillofacial, dental and ENT screen	
	with appropriate treatment	
	stimulation – TENS, acupuncture	Chapter 4
	nerve block	Chapter 5
psychology	stress management, rehabilitation	Chapter 6

CHRONIC PANCREATITIS

pharmacology	simple analgesics	Chapter 3
	NB opioids increase sphincter pressure	
	increase pain	
physical	celiac plexus block	
	spinal drug delivery	Chapter 5
	stimulation – TENS	Chapter 4

b) Behavioural Pain

Behavioural pain can be regarded as a variation of chronic nocigenic pain which has developed beyond the stage where analgesia is possible and where the change to chronicity is associated
with changes in the interpretation of the pain message and the
development of pain behaviours. Treatment is directed towards
the patients distress and not by the pain. The main thrust of pain
management is the psychological elements of re-education and
behavioural modification coupled with appropriate physical
therapy advice. Individual additional components may be necessary as indicated below.

Analgesic Summary

Pharmacological	Antidepressants	Chapter 3
Psychological	Cognition	Chapter 6
	Behaviours	
Physical	Functional Therapy	Chapter 7
	General Fitness	
	Stimulation analgesia	Chapter 4
	Spinal analgesia	Chapter 5

Examples:

FACIAL PAIN

pharmacology	antidepressants	Chapter 3
physical	acupuncture	Chapter 4

SPINAL PAIN (LOW BACK, NECK)

pharmacology	antidepressants	Chapter 3
	capsaicin	
physical	stimulation – TENS, SCS, Acupuncture	Chapter 4

ABDOMINAL PAIN (IRRITABLE BOWEL, CHRONIC PELVIC PAIN)

physical	sympathetic block	Chapter 5
stimulation	TENS	Chapter 4

NON–ANGINAL CHEST PAIN

physical	stimulation – TENS	Chapter 4

FIBROMYALGIAS

pharmacological	antidepressants	Chapter 3
physical	stimulation –- acupuncture	Chapter 4

REPETITIVE STRAIN INJURY

physical therapy	retraining in appropriate skill

COMPLEX REGIONAL PAIN DISORDER (REFLEX SYMPATHETIC DYSTROPHY)

a) early phase:		
physical therapy	desensitisation functional therapy	Chapter 7
physical	nerve block for desensitisation	Chapter 5
b) end stage:		
physical	spinal analgesia – clonidine	Chapter 5
	stimulation – SCS	Chapter 4

c) Neurogenic Pain

Neurogenic pain does not arise by stimuli activating the classical pain pathways. Neurogenic pain occurs in the absence of an adequate stimulus. Because of these two factors chronic neurogenic pain does not, in general, respond to either analgesics or anatomical blocking. The exceptions being trigeminal neuralgia and spinal cord injury, including nerve avulsion. Acute neurogenic pain may respond to nerve blocks and analgesics. The pain is often unremitting and is associated with significant depression.

Analgesic summary

Acute Neurogenic Pain		
Pharmacology	According to the analgesic staircase	Chapter 3
Physical	Nerve Blockade	Chapter 5
Chronic Neurogenic Pain		
Pharmacology	Antidepressants Anticonvulsants	Chapter 3
Physical	Desensitisation	Chapter 7
	Stimulation	Chapter 4
Trigeminal Neuralgia		
Pharmacology	Carbamazepine +/- baclofen	Chapter 3
Physical	Rhizotomy/ microvascular decompression	Chapter 5
Spinal Cord Injury/Nerve Avulsion		
Physical	DREZ Cordotomy	Chapter 5

Examples:

POSTHERPETIC NEURALGIA

acute phase:		
pharmacology	analgesic staircase	Chapter 3
physical	regional nerve block	Chapter 5
chronic phase:		
pharmacology	tricyclic antidepressant	Chapter 3
	capsaicin	
physical	regional blockade if hyperaesthesia present	Chapter 5
	TENS, Acupuncture	Chapter 4

PERIPHERAL NERVE INJURY

acute phase:		
pharmacology	analgesic staircase	Chapter 3
	steroids	
	antidepressants	
physical	proximal nerve block	Chapter 5
	surgical decompression if required	
chronic phase:		
pharmacology	antidepressants	Chapter 3
	anticonvulsants	
physical	stimulation – TENS, SCS	Chapter 4
	desensitisation	Chapter 7
	sympathetic nerve block	Chapter 5
	assessment for DREZ	

A particular form of pain after peripheral nerve injury is Complex Regional Pain Disorder type 2, previously known as **Causalgia**. In this condition there is marked autonomic hyperactivity in association with chronic burning pain. Treatment includes both temporary and neurolytic sympathetic blocks.

PHANTOM PAIN

pharmacology	antidepressants	Chapter 3
	anticonvulsants	
physical	stimulation – TENS, SCS, Acupuncture	Chapter 4
	sympathectomy if 'cramping' evident	Chapter 5

With phantom pain there is often a need to change treatments regularly.

NEUROMA

pharmacology	anticonvulsants	Chapter 3
physical	desensitisation	Chapter 7
	local or neurolytic blockade	Chapter 5
	excision	

CENTRAL POST-STROKE PAIN

pharmacology	antidepressants	Chapter 3
	anticonvulsants	
physical	desensitisation	Chapter 7

CENTRAL SPINAL CORD PAIN

pharmacology	antidepressants	Chapter 3
	anticonvulsants	
physical	stimulation – SCS	Chapter 4
	spinal drug delivery – opiates,	
	clonidine, baclofen	Chapter 5
	surgical – cordotomy, cordectomy	

TRIGEMINAL NEURALGIA

pharmacology	anticonvulsant – carbamazepine;	
	second line baclofen	Chapter 3
physical	rhyzolysis – radiofrequency, phenol,	
	glycerol, alcohol	Chapter 5
	neurosurgical – microvascular	
	decompression	

d) Psychogenic Pain

Psychogenic pain is very rare, there has often been an experience of nocigenic or neurogenic pain. The diagnosis must be made using positive indicators of psychiatric illness. Hysterical pain, Munchhausen's syndrome and delusional pain all occur and require appropriate management. The diagnosis should not be made on grounds of exclusion. Drug seeking behaviour may also manifest as a pain complaint especially when opiate drugs have been given inappropriately.

Examples:

HYSTERICAL PAIN

Various features may be present including the dependent histrionic personality type. Pain is often described in simple sensory terms. Pain does not arouse the patient from sleep. There is often excessive analgesic use. Complaints of depression are common.

AFFECTIVE DISORDERS

There is a close association between chronic pain and depression. Occasionally, however endogenous depression may present with pain and frequently suicidal ideology. This is a psychiatric emergency.

PSYCHOTIC DISORDERS

The patient may present with delusional pain. This is often severe and persistent in one body area and may not be 'bizarre'. There may be self mutilation as an attempt to stop the pain. Interestingly acute pain sensitivity is diminished in schizophrenia.

Particular Pain Problems

Spinal pain

Pain may arise in a single spinal segment – cervical, thoracic or lumbar – or in a combination of sites. Certain warning signs or 'red flags' may be present which require urgent assessment by orthopaedic or neurosurgeons. These include age <20 and >55, a history of significant trauma, systemic symptoms such as weight loss, drug use and abuse, progressive non-mechanical pain, severe mechanical restriction, widespread neurology and structural deformity.

Radicular pain

Nerve root distribution of pain with or without spinal pain requires early referral and investigation since some cases may be surgically remedial. The pain may arise due to trauma, prolapsed intervertebral disc infection, arteritis, tumour, or by degenerative changes. There may be demonstrable numbness or paraesthesiae in the same distribution. Movements which stretch the affected nerve root elicit pain, for example straight leg raise or femoral stretch. Pain in prolapsed intervertebral disc is aggravated by flexion. Prognosis in cases such as prolapsed disc is reasonable with 50% recovering from an acute attack within six weeks. Treatment is as for neurogenic pain as described above.

Cauda equina syndrome

This is often associated with difficulty in micturition and loss of sphincter tone. There may be saddle anaesthesia and widespread multiple root involvement with weakness in the legs. This is a surgical emergency requiring immediate referral as some cases may be reversible.

Inflammatory disorders

An example is ankylosing spondylitis. This presents with a gradual onset with morning stiffness. There is progressive limitation of spinal movement in all planes. There may be other connective tissue symptoms and signs and a positive family history. The patient should be referred to a rheumatic disorders specialist. Treatment consists of appropriate analgesics including TENS and exercise.

Referred visceral pain

Oesophageal, pericardial and aortic disease may produce pain referred to the thoracic spine. Aortic, gastro-duodenal, pancreatic, renal diseases and mesenteric ischaemia may all produce pain referred to the lumbar spine. These conditions require exclusion from the differential diagnosis with treatment of the underlying condition.

Vertebral element pain

Conditions affecting the zygapophyseal joints may affect all spinal levels. The pain is typically aggravated by spinal extension. The condition may be diagnosed by selective local anaesthetic blockade. Facet joint pain may produce referred radicular pattern pain. In the cervical spine pain can arise from the alar ligament. In the thoracic spine pain can arise from the costal joints and costotransverse ligaments. These can be localised by selective injections. Management consists of simple analgesics, and TENS.

Muscle origin pain

This may be associated with trigger points, muscle spasm or be dysfunctional pain. The pain is typically paraspinal but may produce a referred pain pattern. It is important to exclude treatable causes such as infective processes and neoplasm. The conditions may arise because of concomitant spinal pathology, for example trauma or degeneration.

Treatment of trigger point and muscle spasm pain may include trigger point injections or acupuncture. These muscular origin pains often require use of low dose tricyclic antidepressants and progressive exercise programme or pain management programme.

Headache

There are several recognisable headache conditions which may require specific treatments.

Migraine

This may present as 'Classical Migraine' with aura or without aura. The classical form is typically preceded by a prodrome or aura with nausea, vomiting and photophobia. It is typically unilateral and throbbing in character. There may be precipitating factors such as stress or dietary factors.

Treatments consist of ergot preparations, B-blockers, calcium blockers, NSAIDs and sumatriptan. Exclusion of precipitating factors may be important. Prophylaxis by B-blockers and calcium blockers. Chapter 3

Carotidynia

Throbbing pain in the neck radiating into the face. May be precipitated or aggravated by head movement, coughing or swallowing. The carotid arteries may be tender on palpation.

Treatments and prophylaxis as for migraine. Chapter 3

Cluster Headache

Unilateral facial pain occurring in bouts or clusters. Associated with lacrimation, nasal stuffiness conjunctival injection and photophobia. May be aggravated by alcohol and stress. May occur as a chronic cluster headache, particularly in men, which can be less amenable to treatment.

Treatment consists of ergot preparations, calcium blockers, NSAIDs, sumatriptan and oxygen. Chapter 3

Chronic Paroxysmal Hemicrania

Daily unilateral facial pain associated with head movement more common in females. May have autonomic signs in the face and occasionally tinnitus, facial hypersensitivity and extrasystoles. This may occur as a chronic unremitting or as a remitting variety depending on temporal characteristics.

Treatment by NSAIDs particularly indomethacin Chapter 3

Cluster-Tic Syndrome

This is a coexistence of a chronic cluster pattern of pain with trigeminal neuralgia which may occur in middle age.

Treatment by carbamazepine or baclofen Chapter 3

Syndrome of Jabs and Jolts

Also known as ice-pick headache. Intermittent short stabs of pain which may be aggravated by neck movement. Usually self

23

limiting but may respond to NSAIDs such as indomethacin.

Chapter 3

Temporal Arteritis

Throbbing temporal pain occurring often after the fifth decade. May be aggravated by eating. There may be accompanying visual disturbance from the arteritis.

Treatment is by corticosteroids and immunosuppressants.

Low Cerebrospinal Fluid Pressure and Post–dural puncture headache

Dull, aching or throbbing headache aggravated by standing up and relieved by lying down. There may be neck stiffness dizziness or tinnitus and blurred vision. This may arise spontaneously or following dural puncture.

Treatment consists of NSAIDs, adequate hydration, epidural injection of blood (Blood Patch)

Tension Headache

Pain over the scalp often associated with pain radiating into the neck. May be described as a tight band around the scalp. Associated stress and tension.

Treatment consists of simple analgesics and stress reducing techniques.

Pain in Children

The principles of pain management for adults is the same for children with a few additional features:

a) Pain report and measurement

   This is more difficult to ascertain. The quiet child may be more distressed but withdrawn. Children may be unable to explain what they feel and behavioural signs become invaluable.

b) Pharmacology

   Appropriate dosage per body mass is required. (Table 3)

c) Techniques

   Most techniques used in adults have been used in appropriate cases in children. Physical interventions may be less well tolerated due to procedural pain and may need to be implemented under sedation or even light general anaesthesia. Stimulation techniques such as acupuncture and TENS can be used.

d) Prognosis.

Certain problems 'burn out' with time, for example juvenile rheumatoid arthritis. Other problems, for example complex regional pain disorder (RSD), carry a worse prognosis in children than in adults.

Drug	Dose mg/kg	Route	Frequency (hrs)
Paracetamol/ Acetaminophen	10-20	o/pr	4-6
Aspirin	10-20	o	4
Ibuprofen	5-15	o/pr	6-8
Naproxen	5-7	o	8-12
Morphine	0.1-0.3	o/pr	4-8
Codeine	0.75-1.5	o	4-6
Methadone	0.1-0.4	o	24
Imipramine	3-5 mg/kg/day	o	24
Amitriptylene	3-5 mg/kg/day	o	24

Table 3 – Common paediatric drugs and doses

Pharmacology

Pharmacokinetics

Before considering individual drugs it is relevant to briefly consider pharmacokinetics. With most agents a certain plasma concentration of agent is necessary to get a sufficient concentration into the tissue phase where it is needed. Variations in solubility in the various tissue components and the addition of substances which may delay or in some cases increase absorption may all influence the speed of onset, the duration and the speed of offset of drug action. Adverse effects and side effects may also depend on the same factors. Drug metabolism is also of importance both in relation to the offset of action by metabolism and excretion of the drug, but also in relation to prodrugs, for example the metabolism of codeine to morphine.

Drugs administration is commonly divided into enteral, that is via the gastrointestinal tract, and parenteral, that is all other methods. The advantage of the enteral routes is that the bodies infection barriers are not breached reducing the possibility of treatment failure by infection. There are two types of enteral administration depending on whether the agent passes through the portal tract or not. These are the conventional oral method which contrasts with the bypass routes which include buccal, sublingual, rectal and vaginal administration. The parenteral routes include transdermal and inhalational routes in addition to those requiring needles such as subcutaneous and intradermal, intramuscular, intravenous and spinal routes.

Enteral

a) Oral

The drug is swallowed or administered through an intestinal tube and absorption takes place through the gastrointestinal tract. Drug may be given as a tablet or in the form of a liquid depending on what the patient can consume.

Absorption may be pH dependent. Aspirin is least polar in the stomach and is absorbed there. In contrast paracetamol (acetaminophen) is insoluble in the stomach and is wholly absorbed from the small intestine. In consequence the onset of aspirin is faster than paracetamol. Other drugs may be actively taken from the intestinal tract by carrier mechanisms.

Absorption from the intestinal tract is over a period of time as the agent passes along the gut. This transit may be altered by the co-administration of drugs which may increase or slow gut transit, for example opiates slow gut transit times. In addition the drug may be altered or encapsulated to delay its absorption.

Drugs absorbed from the gut first enter the portal venous system and pass through the liver. With some drugs, for example morphine, there is a significant 'first pass' hepatic uptake such that only one third of the administered drug enters the systemic circulation. With other drugs, such as buprenorphine, so much drug is destroyed in this way that oral administration is futile.

b) Buccal, Sublingual, Rectal, Vaginal
Venous drainage of the oral cavity, rectum and vagina is directly into the systemic veins avoiding transhepatic passage and loss of the 'first pass' effect. This allows a more rapid access to the systemic circulation as well as allowing an enteral route of administration of a drug which could not be given orally. Care is needed with the buccal and sublingual route that the patient does not swallow the drug solution which may result in treatment failure. With the rectal and vaginal route care is needed that the patient does not lose the drug before it is absorbed.

Parenteral
a) Inhalational
Drug entering the tracheobronchial tree is absorbed rapidly through the respiratory mucosa with rapid access to the arterial system. This route is used to administer the anaesthetic volatile agents and the analgesic gas nitrous oxide. The less soluble the agent, as with nitrous oxide, the more rapidly it equilibrates with plasma and hence with the nervous system. This allows for very rapid analgesic onset, and offset, of action.

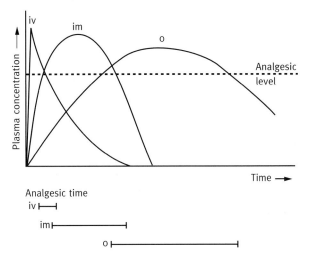

Figure 1 – Pharmacokinetics and analgesic 'time' for intravenous (iv), intramuscular (im) and oral (o) administration

Intranasal administration is used to allow administered drug to gain access to the respiratory mucosa in the upper airway. The hormone calcitonin has been given this way to avoid administration by injection.

b) Transdermal
Drugs applied to the skin may be absorbed slowly. The drug molecules have to be small enough and soluble enough to be absorbed through intact epidermis. Onset of action is therefore very slow. Once the drug has been absorbed into the dermal layers it cannot be removed. This creates a potential problem for overdose and toxicity. Drugs administered this way include the opioid fentanyl, the alpha agonist clonidine, capsaicin and the local anaesthetics.

c) Intradermal/subcutaneous
Injection of drug into the dermis, or just through the dermis into the subcutaneous tissues. Absorption is slow from these sites as with transdermal administration and once administered

drug cannot be withdrawn. There is slow steady absorption from particularly the subcutaneous site allowing this to be use for continuous infusion. Spread of absorption can be decreased using vasoconstrictors and increased using hyaluronidase. Problems occur with inflammation and infection with long term use. It is however relatively 'low-tech' being easy to replace indwelling needles allowing rotation of infusion sites.

d) Intramuscular

Injection of drug into a muscle belly produces a peak plasma concentration between 15 and 30 minutes. This can be delayed by using vasoconstrictors or by preparing sustained release or depot preparations. Once administered drug cannot be withdrawn which may produce problems with overdose. Skill is required for administration to avoid damaging other structures, for example nerves, and to avoid vascular injections. It is not a site for continuous administration since needles and catheters will move with the underlying tissues.

e) Intravenous

Intravenous injection of drug allows instant access to the vascular component with rapid entry into the tissues. Due to the relatively preferential perfusion of the central component of nervous system and cardiovascular systems there is rapid onset of action with higher peak concentrations than with the intramuscular route. There is also be a rapid decline in plasma concentrations due to redistribution.

Various strategies are available to allow continuous administration to achieve more stable plasma concentrations using pumps or syringe drivers. Continuous intravenous infusion is one such. An alternative is Patient Controlled Analgesic infusion. Continuous infusion allows a continuous plasma concentration to be achieved but may be associated with overdosage when used for longer periods as drug accumulation occurs. This is particularly the case when other medical conditions may affect metabolism and excretion. Patient controlled analgesic infusions were developed to allow small repeated boluses to be administered. These multiple mini-peaks create an almost steady state but allow the concentrations to fall between each peak. If relative overdosing occurs then patient demand will fall and the concentration will fall. This requires sophisticated apparatus with safeguards to prevent or minimise interference with dosing or dangerous surges of medication.

Short duration intravenous administration may be easily given via a peripheral vein. For longer duration administration cannulation of a central vein with tunneled or implanted catheters is essential to secure access and to reduce the incidence of infection. Safety of dosing and infection are the largest problems with intravenous administration.

f) Spinal

Drugs may be administered into the spinal canal into either the extradural or intradural (subarachnoid) spaces. These routes allow the delivery of small doses of drugs close to the site of action in the spinal cord thereby minimising the systemic dose of drug and its side effects. The spaces can be catheterised using temporary percutaneous catheters or using sophisticated implanted pump technology. Extradural administration produces some systemic drug action, with plasma levels approaching an intramuscular profile, and catheters are prone to blockage by fibrosis. Intradural catheters use smaller doses and are less prone to blockage.

Analgesics

Drugs which have a primary analgesic action may belong to one of several categories. These are the simple analgesics, the opioid analgesics and the Non-Steroidal Anti-Inflammatory analgesics. There is the analgesic NMDA antagonist ketamine, the substance P depletor capsaicin, the peptide somatostatin and the adrenergic agonist clonidine. There are also miscellaneous drugs which have been used as analgesics in for example rheumatoid arthritis which do not belong to the above groups.

Analgesic Staircase

The different analgesic groups have increasing potencies and may be thought of in terms of a series of steps – the so-called analgesic staircase. This consists of the simple analgesics on the lowest level – principally paracetamol/acetaminophen. The compound analgesics form the intermediate level (table 4) together with some of the 'weaker' opioids. The highest level consists of the strong opioids. In the treatment of cancer pain and acute pain when the agents of one level are ineffective it is appropriate to move up the staircase. Similarly in acute pain steps down should be taken rather than abruptly stopping all analgesics.

(I) Continuous infusion

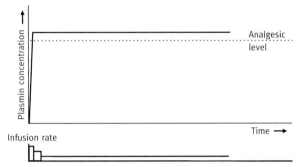

(II) Patient controlled analgesia (PCA)

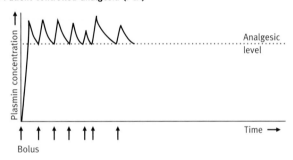

(III) Sustained release oral

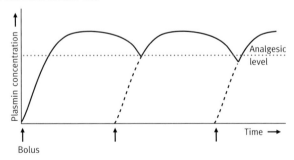

Figure 2 – Pharmacokinetics and analgesic 'level for continuous delivery - infusion, PCA and sustained release oral

The NSAIDs can be used to synergistically augment the analgesics in the staircase. Use of some of the non-analgesics may also allow a reduction in steps or a reduction of dose of the primary analgesic.

Simple analgesics
PARACETAMOL/ACETAMINOPHEN
This drug is used as a sole analgesic or combined with opioids (see table 4).

Use:
Mild to moderate pain as tablet or solution.
Dose in adults 500-1000mg 4 hourly, in children 10-15 mg/kg 6 hourly

Complication:
Lethal hepatotoxicity in overdose.

NEFOPAM
A simple analgesic with cholinergic properties. Given orally or sublingually is approximately 1/3 potency of morphine.

Use:
Mild to moderate pain as tablet.
Dose 10mg 4-6 hourly

Complications:
Tachycardia and sedation.

Opioid analgesics
There is a wide array of opioids with confusing divisions into agonists/antagonists and by receptor type. There is a range of drug actions and formulations range from oral, buccal, sublingual, rectal, injectable or transdermal routes (see Table 5). Certain 'weak' opioids are used in combination with paracetamol. Morphine is the classical drug and many of the other opioids – dihydromorphine, codeine, oxycodone – are pro-drugs, being metabolised to morphine or contain morphine, as in papaveretum. Synthetic opioids derived from pethidine/meperidine and fentanyl are of more use in anaesthetic practice.

There is no 'maximum dose' for most of the direct acting opioids. Side effects may occur to limit the tolerated dose. There is no set dose at which side effects occur. There may be a ceiling effect to analgesia for a drug such as buprenorphine which is a partial agonist.

In the treatment of patients with for example cancer pain it is important to give a reasonable starting dose of drug, for example 30 to 60 mg to the opioid naive patient and to use effective dose increments, increasing by 30 to 50% at each step rather than by slow small increments. If the patient suffers from drowsiness or other side effects the dose should be tapered back. It is important to administer the opioid in regular intervals to try and prevent breakthrough pain.

If using opioids do give an effective dose with effective dose increments. Do not give subcutaneous infusions or fentanyl patches simply because the patient has a diagnosis of cancer – oral morphine is well tolerated and should be used while the patient can take oral medication. Do not mix opioids particularly with reference to breakthrough medication – give the patient a small dose of the maintenance drug to take. Do not use mixed agonist antagonist or partial agonist drugs – they have no advantages over the straight agonists.

There are several useful conversion approaches in addition to that in Table 5, which shows the conversion factor to obtain equivalent analgesia with oral morphine. Calculation of the new opioid dose:

$$\frac{\textit{Equianalgesic dose and route current drug}}{\textit{24 hour dose current drug}} = \frac{\textit{Equianalgesic dose and route new drug}}{\textit{24 hour dose new drug}}$$

Conversion of oral to parenteral:
Morphine Oral 3mg = Oral Diamorphine 2mg = Parenteral Morphine 1.5mg sc. = Parenteral Diamorphine 1mg = Parenteral Hydromorphone 0.2mg

Uses:
Severe pain. Cancer pain. Some nocigenic chronic pain. Acute pain. Anti-tussive.

Complications:
Respiratory depression. Nausea and vomiting. Constipation. Sedation. Paradoxical pain. Addiction.

Tramadol Dose 100mg oral or by injection, 6 hourly
This is a novel analgesic with Mu-opioid receptor activity with
a ceiling effect. It is an adrenergic and serotonergic uptake
blocker. It is claimed to be potent with 100mg = 10mg morphine. It is claimed to be non-addictive.

Uses:
Moderate to severe pain

Side effects:
Agitation and restlessness. Nausea. Seizures. Addiction has been
reported.

Non-Steroidal Anti-Inflammatory Drugs
These drugs act by inhibiting prostaglandin and cyclooxygenase
production both in the periphery and in the central nervous system. There is a wide array of drug types (see Table 7) in different chemical classes. If a certain class of NSAID is ineffective it
may be worth changing to another group. There is a range of
potencies with indomethacin and diclofenac at the most potent
end of the spectrum. Longer acting preparations are available for
some types and a variety of formulations including oral, rectal
and injectable. Gel formulations are available for benzydamine,
piroxicam, diclofenac and felbinac, but significant absorption
can occur. With NSAIDs use one at a time – mixing agents
confers no advantages and may speed the onset of problems.
Remember NSAIDs are not muscle relaxants. Also remember
creams are absorbed and all forms may affect the gastrointestinal
tract – you do not have to take the drug orally to get ulcers!

Uses:
Moderate to severe pain. Inflammatory and postoperative pain.

Complications:
Gastric ulceration. Bronchospasm. Renal dysfunction. Bleeding
tendency due to platelet dysfunction. Allergy. Idiosyncratic
reactions including fixed drug reactions and blood dyscrasias.

NMDA Active: **Ketamine** Dose 0.5-1.0mg/kg iv.
This is a phencyclidine derivative drug developed as a dissociative general anaesthetic. In low doses is analgesic. It is under
investigation for some types of chronic pain, although severe
side effects so far preclude its use.

Use:
Acute pain.

Complication:
General anaesthesia. Dissociative psychomimetic effects not well tolerated.

Capsaicin
This is a substance P depletor which is naturally occurring in red chili pepper. It is use transdermally as a cream in 0.25–0.75% solution.

Uses:
Postherpetic neuralgia. Arthritis pain. Scar pain. Has been used intranasally for cluster headache.

Complications:
Burning pain and heat hyperalgesia may not be tolerated.

Peptide: Somatostatin
Octreotide Dose 50 μg twice daily, up to 600 μg a day in carcinoid syndrome.

This gastrointestinal peptide hormone has been used by infusion and spinally. Octreotide is a synthetic octapeptide.

Use:
Used to control gastrointestinal disturbances.
End stage cancer pain not responding to opioid.

Complications:
Gastrointestinal symptoms, myalgia, backache, anxiety and irritability. May be neurotoxic.

Adrenergic drug: **Clonidine**
This alpha2 adrenergic partial agonist has been used both orally, transdermally and by injection in the treatment of pain.

Uses:
Orally 25-50 μg twice daily for headache. Transdermal patches have been used to desensitise neuropathic areas. Intraspinal use 75-300 μg per day used in neuropathic pain.

Complications:
Hypotension and bradycardia. Sedation.

Anti-Rheumatoid drugs
A variety of anti-inflammatory agents have been used in Rheumatoid arthritis, for example sodium aurothiomalate and penicillamine. A standard Rheumatology text should be consulted for further information.

Non-analgesics

Several drugs are used in chronic pain patients to augment other treatments in an attempt to reduce distress. These drugs have no primary analgesic action.

Tricyclic antidepressants

Tricyclic antidepressants appear to reduce pain complaint in patients with chronic pain. There are three possible mechanisms of action. First, they are antidepressants and depression is present in many chronic pain states. Secondly, they are sedating agents. This may help in two ways namely that if the patient is slightly sedated they may not notice the pain as much, in addition they act as hypnotic such that if the patient sleeps better they are more able to cope the next day. Thirdly, it has been shown in patients who are also taking opioid drugs the bioavailability of opioid is increased by the antidepressant. The tricyclic drugs are membrane stabilising which may account for the early onset of action in chronic pain patients.

The most effective drug is amitriptylene. In patients who are less tolerant of the sedation other tricyclics such as desipramine may be better tolerated. In children imipramine has been used most often and may be the drug of choice.

Dosage:
Amitriptylene 25 to 150 mg daily in divided doses
Desipramine 25 to 100mg daily in divided doses
Nortriptylene 12.5 to 50mg daily in divided doses
Dothiepin 25 to 150 mg daily in divided doses
Imipramine In children 0.2 gradually rising to 3 mg/kg. In adults 20-100 mg daily

Uses:
Central pains such as postherpetic neuralgia, central post-stroke pain, phantom pain, diabetic neuropathy. Other pain problems include fibromyalgias, atypical facial pain, low back pain, any pain with depression.

Contraindications/Side effects:
Glaucoma, Urinary retention, constipation, orthostatic hypo-tension, sedation and dry mouth.

Other Antidepressants

Many of the other antidepressants have been used in patients with chronic pain, particularly when side effects or contraindications preclude the use of the tricyclic antidepressants. No other class of agents has achieved the efficacy of the tricyclics but may be needed to treat the co-existing depression.

Anticonvulsants

Several drugs with a membrane stabilising action have been used in patients with chronic pain. The anticonvulsants all act by general central nervous system depression and are all sedating. The cardiac membrane stabilising drugs (below) were introduced in an attempt to minimise the sedation. The new generation of anti-epileptic drugs acting via GABA are under investigation for use in chronic pain but have so far not become established therapy, and may have major side effects.

Uses:
They are used in the treatment of trigeminal neuralgia and other so called neurogenic pains with a lancinating or shooting component. They may be used empirically in other conditions.

Phenytoin Dose up to 200 mg daily in divided doses.

Side effects/Precautions:
Depression. Skin rashes. Gum hyperplasia. Potentiates cimetidine, co-trimoxazole and diazepam.

Carbamazepine Dose up to 1600 mg daily in divided doses. Drug of choice in trigeminal neuralgia.

Side effects/Precautions
Depersonalisation. Not tolerated well by elderly patients. Drug rashes. Bone marrow suppression. Potentiates dextropropoxyphene and cimetidine. Inhibit coumarin anticoagulant action.

Sodium Valproate Dose up to 1200 mg daily in divided doses. Better tolerated as less sedating.

Side effects/Precautions
May cause hepatic dysfunction.

Clonazepam Dose up to 2 mg daily in divided doses. Typical benzodiazepine.

Side effects/Precautions:
Like other benzodiazepines is addictive in chronic use.

Anti-dysrhythmics

These drugs have been used as an alternative to the antiepileptic drugs in an attempt to reduce the problems with sedation. There has also been interest in developing an oral alternative to lignocaine, which may be analgesic in systemic intravenous doses. This latter phenomenon may however be a manifestation of the cerebral depression of lignocaine rather than a specific activity. Tocainide was used but was associated with exfoliative dermatitis and can no longer be recommended. Flecainide has been used but this drug can cause significant life threatening cardiac dysrhythmias and can no longer be recommended. Current interest centres on mexilitene.

Mexilitine Dose 450-600 mg daily in divided doses.

Use:
Neurogenic pain.

Side effects/Precautions:
Cardiac dysrhythmias.

Vasoactive drugs

These drugs have been used empirically in cases of pain in which vasoconstriction is present including vascular headache

Calcium Channel Blockers

Diltiazam Dose 200-300mg 12 hourly, Sustained release 180-240mg daily
Nifedepine Dose 10mg 8 hourly up to 60 mg day
Verapamil Dose 40-120 mg 8 hourly

Uses:
This class of drug has been used in pain conditions in which vasoconstriction has been thought to play a role for example vascular headache. Also used inappropriately in so called RSD.

Side effects:
Heart failure, bradycardia, dyspnoea, oedema, rashes, dizziness, diarrhea, flushing.

B-blockers

Propranolol Dose 80mg rising to 240 mg daily, divided or slow release.

Uses:
Conditions in which vasoconstriction is implicated for example vascular headache. Also used for its anxiolytic effects.

Side effects:
Cold extremities, heart failure, bradycardia, depression.

Ergot Alkyloids
Ergotamine Dose divided up to maximum 6mg in 24 hours, 10 mg in 7 days.

Uses:
Migraine headache

Side effects:
Vasoconstriction. Angina.

Serotonergic
Sumatriptan Dose 6mg by injection, maximum twice in 24 hours

Use:
Migraine headache

Side effects:
Vasoconstriction, angina, hypersensitivity, flushing, altered sensation.

Neuroleptics:
Methotrimeprazine Dose 80mg daily in divided doses by IM or SC administration

Uses:
Adjunct to opioids in palliative care both as an anti-nausea agent and for its tranquilizing properties. Has additive analgesic property.

Antihistamine:
Hydroxyzine Dose 450 mg daily in divided doses, parenteral.

Piperazine derivative may act through serotonin or histamine pathways.

Uses:
In palliative medicine as a supplement to opioids. Has useful sedative anti-nausea properties.

Side effects:
Sedation.

Muscle relaxant:
Baclofen Dose up to 100 mg daily in divided doses.

Uses:
Pain states associated with muscle spasticity, for example multiple sclerosis, also used as a second line agent in trigeminal neuralgia.

Side effects and precautions:
May cause drowsiness, nausea and weakness. Problems with peptic ulceration, antihypertensives and in psychoses.

Metabolic drugs:
a) Corticosteroids
Prednisone Dose up to 100 mg daily in divided doses, oral.
Dexamethasone Dose up to 96 mg have been used daily in divided doses, oral or parenteral.

Uses:
These drugs are used in cases of cancer with brain metastases or spinal cord or nerve root compression and in when local tumour invasion of viscera or body wall occurs. Have been used in other cases of nerve compression in smaller doses. Used in inflammatory polyarthropathy. Depot steroids are often added empirically to local anaesthetic solutions.

Side effects:
Common steroid side effects with infection, salt and water balance, hypertension, osteoporosis, diabetogenic, peptic ulceration. Side effects with risk of infection and adrenocortical axis suppression follow the use of injected depot steroids.

b) Calcium metabolism
Bisphosphanates
Etidronate Dose 5-20 mg/kg/day
Uses:
Osteoporosis management, bone pain in cancer, hypercalcaemia.

Side effects:
Allergy, oedema, nausea, diarrhea.

Calcitonin Dose 0.5 mg daily, sc. or im injection

Uses:
Bone pain from osteoporosis or metastatic cancer. Hypercalcaemia. Has been used in the neuraxis (intra-cerebroventricular and spinal subarachnoid space).

Side effects:
Skin rashes, hives, flushing, diarrhea, nausea, chills, dizziness.

c) Other Hormones
Goserelin Dose by depot injection 3.6mg every 28 days.
Synthetic decapeptide.

Uses:
The LHRH analogue goserelin is used in the medical management of hormonally sensitive tumours, for example prostate or
breast, and in the management of mastalgia and certain gynae-
cological disorders such as dysmenorrhoea. Pain associated with
these conditions is reduced with treatment.

Side effects:
With initial therapy a surge of gonadal steroids may occur
resulting in immediate increase in symptoms before suppression. Gonadal suppression. Contraindicated in pregnancy.

Name	Opioid	Other drug
Aspav	Papaveretum 10mg	Aspirin 500 mg
Co-codamol	Codeine 8mg	Paracetamol 500mg
Co-dydramol	Dihydrocodeine 10mg	Paracetamol 500mg
Co-proxamol	Dextropropoxyphene 32.5mg	Paracetamol 325mg
Co-codaprin	Codeine 8mg	Aspirin 400mg
Lorcet	Hydrocodone 2.5, 5 or 7.5 mg	Paracetamol/Acetaminophen 500mg
Lortab, Vicodin	Hydrocodone 5, 7.5 or 10 mg	Paracetamol/Acetaminophen 500mg
Percocet	Oxycodone 5mg	Paracetamol/Acetaminophen 325mg
Roxicodone, Percodan, Tylox	Oxycodone 30mg	Paracetamol/Acetaminophen 325mg

Table 4 – Mixed opioid – paracetamol/acetaminophen/aspirin analgesics

Drug	Brand name	Parenteral Dose (mg)	Oral Dose (mg)	Conversion to Oral morphine	Duration (hours)
Morphine		10	30	1	3-4
Morphine SR	MS Contin, MST	-	30	1	8-12
Diamorphine		5	-	1	3-4
Codeine		130	200	0.08	3-4
Dihydrocodeine			60	0.1	
Dipipanone	Diconal	-	10	0.5	
Dextromoramide	Palfium	-	10	2	1-2
Hydromorphone	Dilaudid	1.5	7.5	7.5	3-4
Oxycodone	Roxicodone, Percocet,				
Proladine		-	30		3-4
Hydrocodone	Vicodin, Lortab	-	30		3-4
Levorphanol	Levo-dromoran	2	4	5	6-8
Methadone		10	20	1	8-24
Buprenorphine		0.3	0.4 (sl)	50	8
Pethidine, Meperidine	Demerol	100	300	0.125	2-3
Meptazinol	Meptid	150	200	0.125	2-3
Nalbuphine	Nubain	10	20	1	3-4
Phenazocine	Narphen	-	5	5	4-6
Pentazocine	Fortral	30	60	0.06	3-4
Fentanyl	Duragesic Transdermal 17µg/hour		-	48-72	

Table 5 – Opioid Analgesics with equianalgesic dose

Morphine dose/ day mg	Morphine dose/ 4 hour mg	Fentanyl dose/ hour mg
100	17	25
220	38	50
390	65	100
750	125	200
1170	195	300

Table 6 – Conversion of oral morphine to transdermal fentanyl

Chemical Class	Drug	Daily dose (mg)	Half-Life (Hours)
Salicylate	Aspirin	3600, divided	15-30
	Alloxprin	6000, divided	15-30
	Benorylate	2000, 12 hourly	15-30
	Diflunisal	500, 12hourly	10-12
	Salsalate	500, 12 hourly	8
Proprionic Acid	Fenbufen	450, 12 hourly	10
	Fenoprofen	600, 6 hourly	2
	Flurbiprofen O/PR	200, 6 hourly	3-4
	Flurbiprofen SR	100, daily	
	Ibuprofen	1600, 6 hourly	2
	Ketoprofen O/PR/IM	200, 12 hourly	2
	Naproxen	750, 8 hourly	12-15
	Naproxen PR	500, daily	
	Suprofen	800, 6 hourly	2
	Tiaprofenic Acid	600, 8 hourly	4-6
Fenamic Acid	Mefenamic Acid	1500, 8 hourly	4-6
	Mefenamic Acid Paediatric	25mg/kg daily	
Phenylacetic Acid	Diclofenac O/IM	150, 8 hourly	1-2
	Diclofenac SR/PR	150, daily	
	Diclofenac Paediatric	2mg/kg daily	
Carboxy and Heterocyclic Acids	Indomethacin	150, 8 hourly	2-5
	Indomethacin PR	300, 8 hourly	
	Sulindac	400, 12 hourly	16
	Tolmetin	1200, 8 hourly	1-5
Enolic Acid	Etodolac	1600, 6 hourly	
Pyrazolones	Phenylbutazone	300, 8 hourly	70
	Azapropazone	1200, 12 hourly	24
Oxicam	Piroxicam O/PR	20, daily	38
	Tenoxicam	20, daily	

Table 7 – Non-Steroidal Anti-Inflammatory Analgesics

Hyperstimulation Techniques

There are several methods of counter-irritation or hyperstimulation techniques many of which are used quite spontaneously without medical prescription. Various non-specific methods such as the use of rubbing or locally applied heat are in common daily use. In addition there are other medically 'approved' methods which will be considered further here.

Acupuncture

There are several related techniques which may be considered together. These include the insertion of fine needles (acupuncture), locally applied pressure (acupressure) and local applied thermal stimulation (moxibustion). Needle stimulation may be superficial just entering the epidermis or can be deeper entering the underlying musculature or periosteum. Each has its advocates. Needling into deeper tissues is associated with a particular sensation called 'dechi'. Problems with acupuncture relate to inserting needles into underlying structures causing visceral injury, pneumothorax, haemorrage, spinal cord injury and the transmission of infection including Hepatitis B and C and HIV virus.

Acupuncture techniques may be applied to the whole body, as in the more classical Chinese form of acupuncture. It may be applied to a particular structure such as the ear, as in auricular acupuncture. A variation of acupressure applied to the soles of the feet is reflexology. Acupuncture techniques can be used in two discrete ways in the management of pain.

a) Counter-irritation acupuncture
In these methods acupuncture stimulation is carried out in the area affected by pain. This is the mechanism of articular

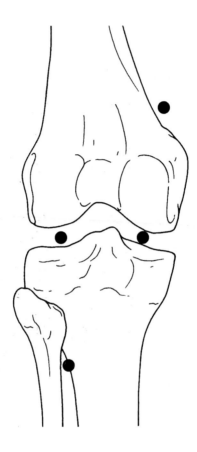

Figure 1 – Acupuncture points for knee pain. Note Joint line points and similarity to intraarticular access for injections

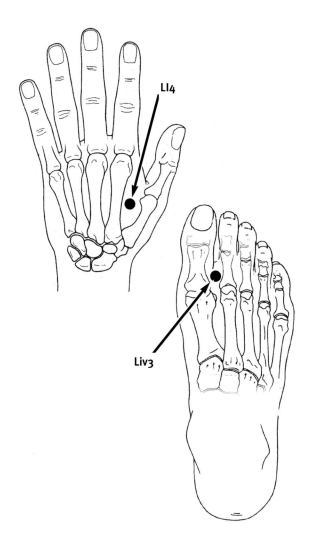

Figure 2 – General acupuncture toning points in the hand (LI4) and Foot (Liv3). Liv3 is also the headache treatment point

acupuncture in which needles are inserted into the periosteum around joints, and is effective in arthritis conditions. A variation of this is the needling of tender areas or trigger points used successfully to treat muscular pain such as low back pain, fibromyalgia, and whiplash pain. Needling or stimulation of the painful structure is followed by relief of symptoms.

b) Relaxation acupuncture

Stimulation of acupuncture points may result in a sensation of relaxation and calm in the patient. In these cases acupuncture may be used to augment relaxation and suggestion methods of pain control. Generalised 'calming' points are in the first web space of the hands (Large Intestine 4) and in the feet (Liver 3).

Electrical Stimulation

Various types of electrical stimulation are used for pain control. There are some common elements. There is an inverse relationship between the frequency of stimulation and the intensity of stimulation which is analgesic. Low frequency stimulation is more likely to recruit motor responses, the ensuing muscular contraction may be painful. Generally stimulation intensity should be such that the stimulation is perceived but is non-painful.

Electrical stimulation techniques are of particular value when there is some degree of nociceptor activation, for example vascular pain, labour pain, cancer pain. Care is needed not to use electrical stimulators during sleep or when using machinery. This is because in the event of an acute disconnection an electrical surge may wake the patient or make them jerk.

a) Transcutaneous electrical nerve stimulation (TENS)

In this method pairs, or multiple pairs, of electrodes are secured on the skin surface. Electrical contact is ensured using gel and the electrode pads secured. Care is needed in selecting electrode sites to avoid stimulation directly over pacemaker generators or the carotid sinus. Most other body sites can be stimulated without difficulty. TENS electrode placement may be at the site of pain or proximally over the trunk or spine. In the initial stages TENS can be used for prolonged periods and the patient needs to explore the best positions for electrode placement and stimulation frequencies and intensities. For obstetric use TENS

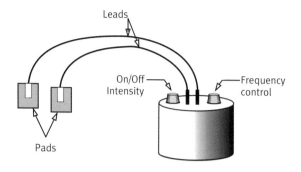

Figure 3 – TENS apparatus showing component parts.

units have a built in higher intensity booster for use during contractions.

TENS apparatus is available 'over-the-counter' and does not require great expertise to apply and use successfully. Problems often seen in patients who have acquired their own stimulators include concern about side effects and contraindications, allergy or sensitivity to the pads, the electrode or more commonly the tape used, help in finding appropriate places for the pads and duration and frequency of stimulation.

A range of alternative pad materials and adhesive dressings may be required. Electrodes may be placed directly over the site of pain, proximally over appropriate nerve tracts and have been placed over acupuncture points. Stimulation frequency may need to be increased or decreased to find the most suitable for the individual. Stimulation may be required for short periods during the day or may be used continuously.

TENS may irritate some patients and low frequency stimulation may cause muscular contractions. This requires a change in frequency delivered. Patients with limited mobility of the shoulders may find it impossible to place electrodes over the spine. If there is no-one to assist this may negate the use of TENS in an individual patient.

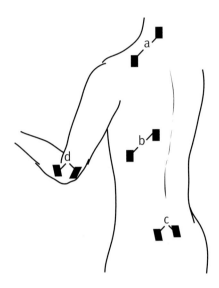

Figure 4 – TENS electrode sites for common pain complaints. a) Brachial plexus and cervical pain, b) intercostal neuralgia, c) lumbosacral pain, d) elbow joint pain.

b) *Transcutaneous spinal electrostimulation (TSE)*

This is a recent development of external stimulation in which electrodes are placed over the spinal cord. The stimulator uses high frequency short pulse width stimulation which is thought to modify descending pain control. Short periods of stimulation can produce long duration analgesia with TSE.

The major problems with TSE are like TENS related to contact sensitivity of the pads. This may require a change in pad or adhesive tape. Some patients may be unable to place the electrodes on themselves. Since there appears to be a prolonged benefit from short periods of stimulation these patients may benefit from attending clinic for the therapy.

c) *Spinal cord stimulation (SCS)*

This was previously known as dorsal column stimulation. In

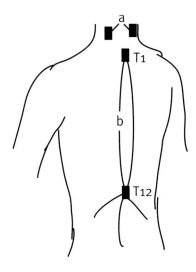

Figure 5 – TSE electrode sites for a) head, neck and arm pain b) other body, spinal pain.

these techniques electrodes are placed in the epidural space over the appropriate spinal cord segments through either a percutaneous needle technique or by laminectomy. The electrode is placed over the appropriate segment and a trial period used to determine feasibility of the technique. If successful the electrode wire is tunneled around the trunk and either connected to an implanted generator or to an aerial. The former is completely self contained and has its own battery supply, the battery needing changing after about five years. In the latter an external battery box stimulator transmits signals which are picked up by the implanted aerial.

Spinal cord stimulation is particularly of value in the treatment of vascular pain. When used for ischaemic limbs or for cardiac pain there is an accompanying improvement in blood flow with treatment. It has also been used to treat complex regional pain syndrome and the so-called 'failed back surgery' syndrome.

The technique has its problems and failure rate with electrode breakage and migration. It also appears to have a decreasing effect with time when used for the non-vascular pains. It is an expensive treatment requiring careful patient selection.

d) Deep brain stimulation (DBS)

In some centres the neurosurgical implantation of electrodes into areas of the brain has been used with success. Electrical stimulation of the pituitary gland has also been used to treat some intractable pain complaints.

Anatomical Techniques

A variety of anatomical techniques are used to disrupt nerve conduction with the desired end point of blocking pain nerves. Several aspects are essential to understanding the why and how of these techniques. Duration of block is central to most of the differences between the different techniques. Disruption can be brought about by chemical, thermal or surgical methods. Different structures may be the target of the block and can be considered in three groups – autonomic, peripheral somatic and central nervous system. Disruption of most peripheral nerves, with the exception of the Trigeminal nerve, produce sensory and motor blockade. Disruption of autonomic nerve may be appropriate for some visceral conditions. Central nerve blocks may allow separation of sensory and motor pathways. Separate consideration should be made of neuromodulation using neuraxial administration of drugs.

In acute pain the assumption made that blocking the nerve produces analgesia holds good. This is not always the case with chronic pain. Many other mechanisms may come into play particularly placebo and nocebo actions. There may also be the role of the systemic absorption of the injected solution which may be 'analgesic'. Differential block using different solutions and placebo may be necessary to confirm the diagnosis and before neurolysis.

Chemical methods
Chemical methods differ with respect to duration of action and reversibility. There is also a group of transdermal medications.

a) Local Anaesthetics
Local anaesthetic drugs produce a reversible block of the action potential of excitable tissues. When this is the axon the desired

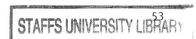

end point – local anaesthesia – results. If this tissue is cardiac or central nervous system then the major side effects – cardiac arrhythmia or convulsions – are the result. Anyone using local anaesthetics must be experienced in the management of these side effects. Duration of local anaesthetic drug is influenced by its physicochemical characteristics (Table 8). Minor prolongation may be obtained by the addition of vasoconstrictor drugs, but these may add to the toxicity and have side effects of their own. Substantial prolongation may be achieved using catheterisation techniques.

Steroids may be added to the local anaesthetic for injection. Controlled studies fail to show significant added benefit from steroid for many regional procedures despite current usage. Intraarticular injection may be an exception.

b) Neurolytic agents

Longer duration neural blockade may be achieved using drugs which damage the nerve axons. The two main agents are phenol and alcohol. Both drugs achieve their end point by dehydrating action by denaturing cell membranes. Both may produce neuritis.

Alcohol in 50 to 100% solutions destroys both axons and the myelin sheath producing long duration analgesia. The predominant disadvantages are severe pain on injection and the high incidence of return of pain into a blocked area (Anaesthesia Dolorosa). This agent has been used to produce somatic nerve block, for example intercostal block. It is used to produce coeliac plexus block. Alcohol solutions are hypobaric compared with cerebrospinal fluid and it may be used to produce neurolytic spinal blockade. Alcohol is also used for pituitary ablation.

Phenol is used in 6 to 10% solution and can be used in aqueous solution or with glycerol Phenol has local anaesthetic properties and is not painful to inject. Its disadvantages include its variable duration of days to months and that it is thrombogenic. Aqueous phenol is used for peripheral nerve block and for lumbar sympathetic blockade. Phenol in glycerol is used to block the trigeminal nerve and because of its hyperbaricity, compared with CSF, to perform intrathecal phenol drops.

c) Transdermal medication

Transdermal application of local anaesthetic using either individual agents or in the eutectic mixture of lignocaine and prilocaine. While predominantly produced to treat acute painful procedures this approach has been used as part of desensitisation of chronic pain and to treat some cases of postherpetic neuralgia. The local anaesthetic needs to be applied to the skin and be absorbed under an occlusive dressing.

Capsaicin, which depletes substance P from nerve fibres can also be used to produce transdermal block of C-fibres. This agent can be rubbed into the painful area and is absorbed through the dermis. It has been successfully used to desensitise chronic pain and to treat postherpetic neuralgia. More recently it has been used to treat pain in arthritis.

Thermal Methods
Both heat and cold can be used to block pain.

a) Cryoanalgesia
Controlled application of low temperatures, down to -70 centigrade, can be achieved using cryoprobes. At these temperatures the axons freeze but the myelin sheath is left intact so that regrowth may occur without neuroma formation. Nerve blockade is produced for several weeks. An iceball is produced in the tissues and may vary from several millimeters to a centimeter in diameter. Direct nerve block may require surgical exposure of the nerve. Cryoanalgesia of painful bony structures, e.g. coccyx or facet joints, is possible by placing the probe against the bone surface.

b) Radiofrequency (heat)
Passing an electrical radiofrequency current through an insulated needle can allow very accurate lesioning of peripheral and central structures. The current produces a controlled tip temperature as desired. This type of lesioning is used in several neurosurgical techniques of pain control.

Surgical techniques
Surgical excision of nerves has been largely superceded by neuromodulation techniques by thermal or chemical methods. Surgical excision of a peripheral nerve produces a neuroma which may be painful or produces a phantom which may be painful. The result is often untreatable neurogenic pain.

Some neurosurgical techniques involving the locating of and the lesioning of central tracts may still have a role in some cases.

Surgical freeing of nerves, for example decompression of the
trigeminal nerve or of trapped spinal nerves, has a role in pain
management. Surgical implantation of drug delivery systems or
stimulators to allow neuromodulation has an increasing role in
chronic pain management. Surgical treatments such as joint
replacement or fixation of traumatic or pathological fractures
also play a significant role it control of pain.

Neuraxial Drug Delivery

One of the major advances of the last two decades has been the
development of long term administration of drugs into the central neuraxis where they may have a more localised action.
These methods are used to modulate pain not to block pain
pathways. If the delivery is stopped then pain returns. Drugs can
be administered intrathecally, into CSF, or extradurally. There
has also been interest in administering drugs into cerebral ven-
tricles. The drug can be administered as a single bolus injection.
This has been used for postoperative pain and to test the effect
of central delivery. Percutaneous and fully implantable systems
have been developed to allow a range of options from repeated
bolusing to constant infusion to multiple variable rate infusions
of drug.

Initially opioids were used and these still remain the mainstay of
central drug delivery. Small doses may produce profound
analgesia without the common side effects of sedation, bowel
slowing, etc. of the systemic drug. The gold standard intrathecal
drug is morphine which has a prolonged duration of action.
Epidurally more lipid soluble drugs such as Diamorphine are
more effective. Careful patient selection including knowledge
that the pain is opioid sensitive but that side effects limit systemic administration is desirable.

Clonidine is the other drug which has repeatedly proven to be
of value. Its role is in the management of neuropathic pain from
spinal cord injury and intractable end stage complex regional
pain syndromes. It needs to be administered in an almost systemic dose and has side effects of drowsiness and cardiovascular
depression.

Baclofen is the other neuraxial drug which has a long term role.
It has greater value in controlling spasticity rather than pain. Its
use is in patients with spinal cord damage who have spasm but

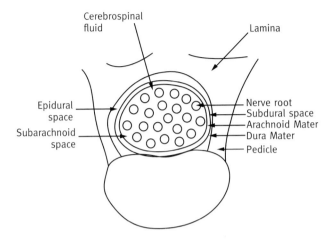

Figure 1 – Spinal compartments. Transverse section at the level of the pedicles.

who cannot tolerate oral baclofen in the required doses.

Indication:
Drug sensitivity but side effects preclude effective dosing.

Complications:
Infection. Catheter failure. Pump failure. Dosage failure. Cost.

Techniques of Regional Blockade

Some methods are within the armamentarium of any medical practitioner whereas other techniques are more demanding and should be available within the practice of pain clinics. It is then useful to know when to refer. With any such technique the practitioner should be versed in resuscitation procedures and be able to deal with side effects and complications.

a) Infiltration and field block procedures
Intradermal and subcutaneous infiltration of dilute local anaesthetic around or in a painful area is used commonly in the acute medical setting but has a limited place in chronic pain.

Indications:
It has been used to infiltrate skin areas involved with herpes zoster, particularly in the subacute stage where it may be of value.

Complications:
Care is needed with total dosage and careful aspiration during injection.

b) Trigger point injections

Many myofascial pain syndromes are associated with the development of 'trigger points' these are present within the muscle bellies. Some chronic postoperative pain conditions are also associated with painful trigger zones. These are often superficial and may even be intradermal but are occasionally deeper. The aim of trigger point injections is to insert the needle point into the trigger point or painful trigger zone. Insertion into a true trigger point is often accompanied by a 'snap' or twitch from the muscle fibres. Injection of a small volume of local anaesthetic solution is all that is often required. Rarely the chronic postoperative scar triggers may require longer blockade using phenol solution or cryoanalgesia.

Indications:
Myofascial pain. Scar pain.

Complications:
Bruising and pain on injection. Intravascular injection.

c) Prolotherapy

This is a variation of trigger point injections used by chiropractors. Injections are made around spinal ligaments and posterior spinal joints using 'sclerosant'. This is an aqueous solution containing both glycerol and phenol. The aim of therapy is the create fibrosis around the ligaments. There is no evidence that this does occur with these trigger points.

Indications:
Myofascial pain, particularly spinal.

Complications:
Bruising, infection and absorption of solution.

d) Ring blocks

Injection of plain local anaesthetic solution on either side of a digit may have a limited role to play in the management of acute episodes of digital pain accompanying arthritic pain.

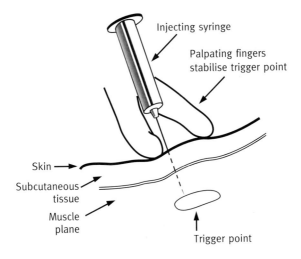

Figure 2 – Trigger point injection into muscle trigger point. One hand fingers stabilise the point for injection

e) Intra-articular blocks

Injection of local anaesthetic solutions into a joint may be of value with acute exacerbations of arthritis pain. One of the many texts on joint injection should be consulted for advice on the exact procedure. Addition of steroid to the solution may not convey any advantages over local anaesthetic alone. In patients with end stage arthritis but who are unsuitable for surgical intervention intraarticular phenol injections have some value.

Indications:
Joint pain.

Complications:
Infection. Joint cartilage trauma.

Specialist regional blocks

Many procedures are available which require special expertise or equipment. It is useful to know what is involved and when to refer.

a) Autonomic blocks

Intravenous regional (sympathetic) block

The intravenous injection of local anaesthetic into a distal vein in a limb which has an inflated proximal tourniquet produces anaesthesia and analgesia of the distal limb. This allows manipulation or desensitisation of the limb to permit functional therapy to take place. There has been a vogue to mix autonomic drugs such as guanethidine, bretylium and reserpine into the solution to produce a 'sympathetic block' but this is unnecessary.

Desensitisation in this way can produce lasting benefit. Joint range can be assessed to allow targeted therapy. A volume of 20-30 ml is required for the arm and from 30-40 ml for the leg, using dilute <0.5% prilocaine or lignocaine which is specially produced for intravenous administration.

Indications:
Persistent limb pain. Particularly with dysfunctional changes.

Complications:
Tourniquet failure with intravascular release of drug. Systemic effects of injected autonomic drugs.

Stellate ganglion block

The cervical paratracheal injection of local anaesthetic solution in order to cover the cervical sympathetic chain. Volumes of 5-10 ml are required to block the head and neck and 10-20 ml to block the arm. Bupivacaine produces a block of only 8-12 hours, Lignocaine for 1 hour

Indications:
This has been used to treat facial and arm pain in acute zoster, phantom arm pain, arm causalgia and some types of facial pain. It has also been used to treat the ocular complications of quinine poisoning. It can be used to assess the potential for thoracic sympathectomy for hyperhidrosis.

Complications:
The technique is associated with many serious complications due to the proximity of the spinal canal and the vertebral artery. Permanent blockade is not recommended.

Thoracic sympathetic block

It is possible to block the thoracic sympathetic chain either percutaneously using local anaesthetic solution or more permanently using radiofrequency coagulation, or under direct

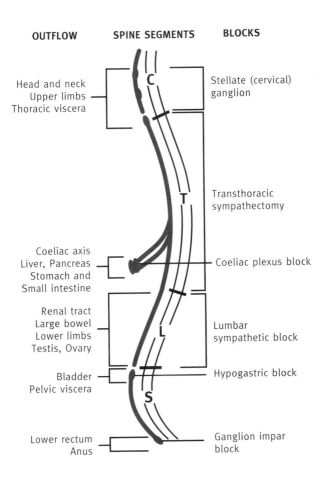

OUTFLOW **SPINE SEGMENTS** **BLOCKS**

Head and neck
Upper limbs
Thoracic viscera

C

Stellate (cervical)
ganglion

T

Transthoracic
sympathectomy

Coeliac axis
Liver, Pancreas
Stomach and
Small intestine

Coeliac plexus block

Renal tract
Large bowel
Lower limbs
Testis, Ovary

L

Lumbar
sympathetic block

Bladder
Pelvic viscera

Hypogastric block

S

Lower rectum
Anus

Ganglion impar
block

Figure 3 – Autonomic nerve block and visceral segments

vision by thoracic endoscopy. Xray screening is mandatory for percutaneous injection. Small volumes of 2-3 ml will produce a block at segmental level.

Indications:
These techniques have been used for upper limb ischaemia, hyperhidrosis and arm causalgia.

Complications:
There is a possible risk of pneumothorax which may need treatment.

Lumbar sympathetic block
Local anaesthetic and neurolytic (5% phenol) solutions can be injected percutaneously onto the lumbar sympathetic chain. Xray screening is mandatory. A volume of up to 5 ml of phenol or local anaesthetic is required. Bupivacaine 0.25% lasts for up to 12 hours. Catheters can be used for longer blocks.

Indications:
These techniques are of value in lower limb ischaemia, leg phantom and causalgic pain and in pain arising from the renal tract, colon and pelvic viscera due to cancer or surgery. Bilateral sympathectomy may be required for some pelvic and other bilateral pains. A low (hypogastric) bilateral block at L5 has been recommended for pelvic pain.

Complications:
Intravascular injection. Thrombosis with phenol has resulted in paraplegia, bowel and kidney infarction. Persistent limb swelling may occur.

Coeliac plexus block
The injection of local anaesthetic or neurolytic (50% alcohol) solutions onto the coeliac axis anterior to the aorta at L1 can be performed. Xray screening is mandatory and some prefer using CT. Volumes of up to 40 ml are used for bilateral procedures using C-arm Xray, smaller volumes have been described when CT scans are used.

Indications:
This is used to treat upper abdominal visceral pain particularly hepatic, oesophagogastric and pancreatic pain from cancer.

Complications:
The neurolytic procedure may produce significant hypotension. Paraplegia has occurred.

Ganglion impar block

Injection of local anaesthetic or neurolytic (5% phenol) solution between the lower rectum and the anterior sacrum blocks the ganglion impar. This is the most caudal autonomic ganglion and supplies the lower rectum. Volumes of up to 1 ml are used.

Indications:
It has been used to treat low rectal and perineal pain.

Complications:
Bowel injury. Infection. Incontinence.

b) Somatic blocks
Trigeminal blocks

The superficial branches of the trigeminal nerve or its ganglion may be blocked using local anaesthetic, neurolytic (5% phenol or 100% alcohol) or thermal methods (cyoanalgesia or radio-frequency) may be used. Ganglion block is intracranial. The exact method will be determined by the type of pain, for example whether due to facial cancer or trigeminal neuralgia, or patient characteristics, for example could they cooperate for sensory testing or not. Xray screening is mandatory. Long duration facial (trigeminal) block can be undertaken with minimal motor impairment. Small volumes of 0.5-1.0 ml are required. 0.5% bupivacaine will last for 8 hours.

Indications:
Trigeminal neuralgia. Cancer pain. Herpes zoster pain.

Complications:
Anaesthesia Dolorosa (return of pain in anaesthetic area) is a risk with some neurolytic procedures. Infection.

Occipital block

The occipital nerve can be palpated, and blocked using local anaesthetic or neurolytic (5% phenol) solutions, where it crosses the superior nuchal line on the occiput. Volumes of 2-3 ml are required.

Indications:
This is useful for posterior head pain due to nerve impingement from for example cervical spondylosis.

Complications:
Haematoma. Infection.

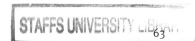

Cervical plexus

Branches from the cervical plexus innervate the ear, the shoulder and the anterior throat. Referred pain to these areas may arise secondary to cervical spondylosis. Local anaesthetic blocks may be of diagnostic value. There is a limited role in chronic pain, but may be of value in neurofibromatosis and cancer pain affecting the cervical roots.

Brachial plexus (including branches)

The brachial plexus may be blocked in the neck, above the clavicle and in the axilla. The choice depends on the expected block. Supraclavicular blocks may block branches to the shoulder and elbow but miss the hand. Infraclavicular blocks miss the shoulder and elbow but are good for the hand. Its branches – radial, median and ulnar nerves – may be blocked at the elbow or at the wrist. For plexus block 30-40 ml of solution are required to fill the neurovascular sheath. Blocks at the elbow require 5-10 ml, while blocks at the wrist require 3-5 ml. Concentration and type of local anaesthetic will depend on the duration and effect desired.

Indications:
Local anaesthetic blockade may have diagnostic value and the plexus may be blocked as a desensitisation procedure for chronic dysfunctional limb pain. Stump pain after amputation. Long term blockade would produce a flail arm disabling the patient, but has been used to treat painful arms after tumour destruction within the plexus.

Complications
Intravascular injection. Spinal spread from interscalene approach. Pneumothorax from supraclavicular approach. Neuropraxias

Intercostal and interpleural block

The chest and abdomen are innervated by segmental intercostal nerves. Local anaesthetic and neurolytic (5% phenol) solutions can be injected either on individual intercostal nerves or several nerves may be blocked using a catheter inserted into the interpleural space. Paravertebral block is when the injection is made proximally adjacent to the vertebral body. If many segments are involved central blocks using either spinal techniques or cordotomy may be more appropriate. A volume of 3-5 ml is required to block an individual intercostal nerve. Interpleural block required volumes of 20-30 ml. A vasoconstrictor is useful due to the high vascularity of the pleura.

Indications:
Body wall pain can arise from tumour invasion of the body wall or pleura. Pain may be referred from the spine and can arise after surgical incisions.

Complications:
Pneumothorax. Intravascular injection. Spinal spread from paravertebral block.

Lumbar plexus block and lower limb blocks

The lumbar plexus and the major trunks – sciatic, femoral, obturator – and the various branches at the knee and ankle may be blocked using local anaesthetic. Long duration blockade, as with brachial plexus, would disable and central blocks may be more appropriate. Volumes of 30-40 ml are required to adequately block the lumbar plexus and to undertake a '3 in 1' block. 25-30 ml are required to block the sciatic nerve, 20 ml to block the femoral nerve and 10 ml to block the obturator nerve at the groin. The tibial, common peroneal and saphenous nerves may all be blocked at the knee and each require 5-10 ml. Branch blocks at the ankle each require 3-5 ml of solution.

Indications:
These may be of value for diagnostic purposes and for desensitisation. Use after amputation for stump pain.

Complications:
Intravascular injection. Neuropraxia.

c) Central blocks
Extradural block

Injection of drugs into the space outside the spinal dura mater using either single bolus injection or the placement of catheters to allow continuous administration of medication. The extradural space can be entered at any level from the cervical spine to the sacral hiatus. The level selected depends upon the site of the pain. Volumes required depend on the level injected with 3-7 ml in the cervical spine, 5-15 ml in the thoracic spine, 20-30 ml in the lumbar spine and 20-30+ ml in the caudal canal.

Indications:
Single injection of local anaesthetic may be of use in spinal pain associated with muscle spasm. The addition of steroid does not

convey any benefit. Injection of neurolytics have been used to treat cancer pain but has been superceded by other techniques, particularly spinal opioid. Continuous extradural drug administration using opioid with or without local anaesthetic drug has an established role in the management of cancer pain and in some other nociceptive pains. Both percutaneous and fully implantable systems are used. Temporary extradural catheters have value in assessing long term spinal drug delivery.

Complications:
Intravascular injection. Intradural injection. Infection. Haematoma.

Intrathecal block

Injection of drugs into the subarachnoid space may be by single bolus or by continuous catheter technique. Continuous spinal catheters can be sited in the lumbar spine because drug spreads freely within CSF.

Indications:
Single bolus of local anaesthetic may be used diagnostically in the investigation of the pain complaint. It has also been used to assess baclofen sensitivity. Intrathecal neurolysis is discussed below. Continuous intrathecal drug delivery of opioid, clonidine and baclofen have established roles in the continuous management of chronic nociceptive pain and spasm.

Complications:
Infection.

Spinal Facet Joint blocks

Back pain may arise from spasm of the posterior spinal muscles aggravated by arthritic changes in the posterior spinal joints. This is often manifested by pain exacerbated by spinal extension. A variation of the technique is injection onto the **Sacro-Iliac Joints** for low back pain aggravated by sacroiliac strain. Injection of local anaesthetic into the posterior joints under Xray control may be therapeutic and diagnostic. In diagnostic cases where the pain returns after the local anaesthetic block terminates longer duration block may be undertaken using cryoanalgesia. Volumes of 1-3 ml are required for facet blocks and 5-10 ml for sacro-iliac. Differential blocks using different agents are essential for facet blocks due to the nature or the responses obtained.

Indications:
Spinal pain exacerbated by extension.

Complications:
Intraspinal spread. Infection

d) Neurolytic procedures
Intrathecal neurolysis

Injection of small volumes of neurolytic solution intrathecally may provide dramatic analgesia in some cases of cancer pain and pain after spinal cord injury. Alcohol (50-100%) is hypobaric whereas phenol (5%) in glycerol is hyperbaric compared with CSF. Dural puncture is performed close to the root origin of the pain and posture used to influence the spread of agent. With alcohol the patient is placed with the painful dermatomes lying above (by gravity) the puncture site. With phenol in glycerol the puncture is performed at L5-S1 with the patient sitting. The phenol is injected and allowed to drop down the CSF to the sacral roots (phenol drop) The techniques have the advantage that they can be performed in the home allowing treatment even late in the terminal phase. Small volumes are used in both techniques, using 0.2-0.5 ml, repeating the procedure at a later date if necessary.

Indications:
Alcohol has a role in body wall pain, for example in mesothelioma. Phenol has a role in patients with perineal pain in whom a 'phenol drop' may be performed and in spinal cord injury in which there is pain below the block.

Complications:
Great care is needed to avoid spread of solution with paralysis and to avoid problems with continence.

Peripheral nerve neurolysis

Peripheral neurolysis has only a limited role because of the accompanying motor block. It may be of value in the terminal cancer patient particularly when nerve infiltration has produced some degree of disability already. Trigeminal neurolysis for facial cancer and trigeminal neuralgia is an exception so too is occipital nerve neurolysis for occipital neuralgia. These have been discussed above.

Cordotomy

Percutaneous cervical cordotomy involves inserting an electrode into the spinal cord at C1-2 using a combination of Xray

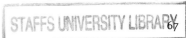

control and sensory testing. The spinothalamic tract can be lesioned producing contralateral analgesia and thermal sensory loss.

Indications:
The ideal patient is one with a limited prognosis of 6-9 months with unilateral pain below C4. Bilateral procedures can be done but need to be staged. In addition to cancer pain it may be of value in spinal cord injury pain and in some other carefully selected cases with nocigenic pain.

Complications:
Problems may occur with breathing when used for chest pain and continence when used for pelvic pain. There is an incidence of ipsilateral weakness in 5-10%.

Pituitary Alcohol neurolysis
Injection of small volumes of alcohol into the pituitary fossa is a technique with limited value having been superceded by LHRH analogues and spinal opioids.

Indications:
There are still some circumstances for which pituitary ablation may be considered, for example in cases with hormonally sensitive tumours (breast or prostate) in whom spinal cord compression is occurring and in cases in whom no other therapy appears to be working.

Complications:
Pituitary failure. Blindness. Persistent CSF leak. Infection.

Neurosurgical Treatments
a) Intracranial procedures
These techniques require the ability to withstand the stress of major surgery and general anaesthesia. They may be unsuitable for the ill and elderly patient.

Microvascular decompression
This is a treatment for trigeminal neuralgia. In this technique the trigeminal roots are identified in their intracranial route and divided from the adjacent vascular structures. The nerve roots are wedged away from the artery which may be responsible for compressing the nerve.

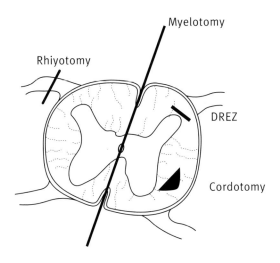

Figure 4 – Neurosurgical spinal cord and root lesioning procedures.

Advantages:
Used for younger fitter patient with trigeminal neuralgia. No nerve damage from the procedure.

Disadvantage:
Craniotomy and its complications.

Thalamotomy
This is surgical disconnection of the sensory thalamus used in extreme cases of intractable cancer pain. It is an intracranial intracerebral procedure.

Disadvantages:
Craniotomy and its complications. Intracerebral surgery and its complications.

b) Spinal Cord procedures
These procedures all have in common the need to be performed with the patient prone through a laminectomy. General anaesthesia is required. Operation on the spinal cord may result in extensive damage, infarction or infection resulting in permanent paralysis or sensory loss.

69

DREZ

In this technique fine electrodes are inserted into the posterior part of the spinal cord where the sensory fibres enter the dorsal area. Fine thermal lesions are created to disrupt small fibre function. This technique is used for deafferentation pain problems.

Uses:
Brachial plexus avulsion. Spinal cord injury associated with nerve root avulsion, e.g. after traumatic paraplegia.

Complications:
Open surgery on the spinal cord. Possible paralysis or major sensory loss. General anaesthesia

Open cordotomy

This is the 'older' method of dividing the spinothalamic tract in the spinal cord under direct vision.

Uses:
Unilateral cancer pain.

Complications:
Open surgery on the spinal cord under general anaesthesia. Paralysis or major sensory loss possible. Return of pain after a period of time due to neuroplasticity.

Midline myelotomy

In this technique the lower part of the spinal cord may be divided in the midline under direct vision. This divides all fibres crossing the midline of the spinal cord producing bilateral spinothalamic tract division. Advantages over cervical cordotomy in that respiratory and autonomic dysfunction may be avoided.

Uses:
Bilateral pelvic pain due to cancer.

Complications:
Open surgery of the spinal cord under general anaesthesia. Division may not be midline interfering with other sensory function.

Cordectomy

This is the surgical transection of the spinal cord with possible excision of the cord. Rarely used to treat intractable pain after spinal cord injury. Requires general anaesthesia in the prone position. May be followed by phantom pain.

Epiduroscopy

Diagnostic endoscopy of the spinal canal is being investigated at present and may offer an alternative to many of the treatments currently used to treat spinal pain.

Drug	Potency	Duration hrs	Clearance l/min	Half-life hrs	Maximum dose
Procaine	2	1	6.56	0.138	
Lignocaine	1	1.5	0.95	1.6	2-5mg/kg
Prilocaine	1	3	2.37	1.6	10mg/kg
Bupivacaine	0.25	4-12	0.58	2.7	2mg/kg
Etidocaine	0.375	4-12	1.11	2.7	6mg/kg

Table 8 – Local anaesthetic drugs in common use

Psychological Approaches

Various psychological techniques are used in the management of pain. Many of these are used spontaneously by individuals in pain. This can be augmented by professional help. In other cases 'abnormal' mechanisms develop and these require professional intervention in order to help the patients to cope better. There are two broad categories within these mechanisms namely cognitive and behavioural. These are not mutually exclusive and can be used to augment each other. The psychological techniques can be used on an individual basis or using group approaches. Important issues are distress, mood and locus of control which are all amenable to psychological intervention.

Cognitive Psychology

Cognitive approaches are based on thoughts, ideas and emotions and their interpretation. The basic aim of therapy is to re-educate the patient in the interpretation of these thoughts, ideas and emotions such that they may be placed in a more appropriate context which will allow the patient to cope. Particular attention is directed to undoing the individuals inappropriate learned pain concepts and behaviours.

Negative thinking
Negative thoughts include, for example, the patient who believes that their back pain is due to cancer. Another common negative thought is that pain always means to rest when in the more chronic pain problems activity is required.

Positive thinking
Patients need help to see the better side of what they think or feel. They need to be able to divert attention to these rather than to their negative thoughts. They need to learn that pain does not

equal invalidity. There is a need to see success with each positive step forward.

Imagery
This is used in processes such as relaxation where the individual uses imagery of warmth and pleasantness to counter negative feelings.

Attention
Some individuals have abnormal sensory awareness. Irritable bowel syndrome is one example where the individual becomes sensitive to normal internal sensation. The patient has to learn how to divert attention away from these feelings. Somatisation may be present in that the patient diverts attention away from external events by concentrating on internal processes, perceiving psychological distress as physical illness.

Behavioural Psychology

Behavioural approaches to pain management are based upon changing what the patient does in such a way that they increase their activities in a purposive way while reducing the impact of the pain.

Pacing and Goal setting

Increased activity is achieved by gradually increasing what is done and achieved thereby preventing failure. Appropriate targets are established to do this and activity paced to gradually increase activity using reward, that is less pain with more gain. Goal setting is crucial to prevent reinjury due to the setting of unrealistic targets and over-exertion. One of the important issues is to break up an activity into smaller components and to concentrate on successfully completing each component rather than an entire activity. Small steps are more important than one large leap. Failure to achieve only serves to reinforce that there is something 'wrong' and that it is acceptable to stop.

Changing activities

It may be important to adopt new activities such as use of relaxation methods or self hypnosis to reduce the impact of pain and stress. In addition there may be negative or abnormal behaviours which may need to be unlearnt. Stopping being active and

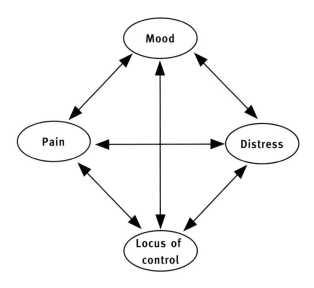

Figure 1 – Interrelationships of pain, mood, control and distress

drug seeking behaviour may need to be modified to allow the individual to cope.

Stress Management

One of the major accompaniments of chronic pain is an increase in stress. Several methods are available to try and relieve some of the stresses and with them the aggravating factors which sometimes drive chronic pain and lead to avoidance behaviour. The patient needs to find a posture in which they can use these relaxation methods. This may be by either lying on a mat, or sitting in a chair.

Relaxation / Breathing
Increasing stress leads to a rise in respiratory rate and reduction in volume. Many stress reducing techniques start with teaching the patient how to breathe in a slow relaxed manner. Breathing techniques teach diaphragmatic breathing and concentrate on

slow deep breathes. The patient is asked to concentrate on feeling expansion of the upper, then middle and then lower parts of the chest during each breath. They then hold the breath for a few seconds before exhaling slowly. During exhalation they are taught to feel the tension lift. Diaphragmatic breathing should be undertaken once or twice an hour during the day.

Deep muscular relaxation
The patient is taught how to contract individual muscle groups and then allow the group to relax before moving onto another area. They should learn a sequence of moves leading to whole body relaxation. For the head they clench the jaws, squeeze the eyes closed and push the tongue against the roof of the mouth then relax. For the forehead and neck they raise the eyebrows high and arch the neck backwards then relax. The hands are clenched then relaxed, then the elbows first flexed and relaxed before extending and relaxing the arms. The shoulders are shrugged high and relaxed. The toes are pointed with legs straight then relaxed. The knees locked in extension and relaxed. The low back is arched and buttocks clenched then relaxed. The stomach held tense then relaxed and finally a deep breath taken and held then relaxed. This sequence can be repeated if the patient still feels tense.

Self Hypnosis
This may be used as an adjunct to the relaxation methods in order to deepen the stress reduction and extend the relaxation. The patient lies down supine in a warm, quiet room. They place their hands on top of each other on their stomach and start by taking deep breaths concentrating on the hands rising and falling. Imagery can be used to augment the sensations. They then breath slowly and comfortably while starting to count down from a number such as 300. As they do so they use imagery or a suggestion tape to held relax, feeling the relaxation extend from the chest down the trunk and along the arms and legs. They concentrate on a feeling of heaviness and warmth traveling along the body areas. Using a combination of suggestion and imagery they are encouraged to feel the body relax into the mat, concentrating on the rhythm of the deep slow breathing and calm thoughts, for example lying on a warm beach. After they relax fully they then count forwards through a short sequence, such as from one to seven, feeling calm and relaxed, opening their eyes on the final count.

Autogenic Relaxation

The patient may learn to use this variant of biofeedback to vasodilate the limbs by concentrating on a feeling of warmth and heaviness. This augments the relaxation techniques. The patient adopts a relaxed posture and takes a few deep diaphragmatic breaths. They then concentrate on each limb in turn, including the shoulders, feeling each become heavy and relaxed, repeated two to three times. There is no active contraction of the muscles. The patient then progresses through a series, feeling each limb to be warm. This is followed by feeling the heart rate to be calm and regular, the breathing calm and regular, the stomach calm and warm and the forehead calm and cool. These feelings are all repeated two to three times in a regular sequence.

Family Therapy

In many chronic pain patients the dysfunction is not just in the individual but may be part of a dysfunctional family or social group. In order to improve the patients functioning it may be important to assess and work with the spouse or significant other, or even the extended family. The social group may have to learn that pain does not mean disability and to concentrate of improving the patients contribution and function rather than reward the pain. In some cases this can be an uphill struggle as a dysfunctional patient may be easier for the family to cope with. The pain 'problem' may be a manifestation of a dysfunctional family.

Other dynamics may be important to explore such as marital disharmony, physical or mental abuse. Past childhood physical or sexual abuse may be relevant.

Multidisciplinary Pain Management

It may prove more expedient to combine psychological and physical approaches together in a multidisciplinary pain program. This type of program centers around improving life skills and reducing distress rather than concentrating on pain. The patients are taught relaxation techniques. They are taught more about the meaning of pain and how to cope with it. They learn to pace activities and set goals and targets. At the same time attention is given to exercise programs and starting to get the patients more active and fitter. They learn that medicine and

surgery cannot cure them and of the side effects and complications of the treatments they use. There is a need to get the
patient to be self caring for the chronic illness and to have an
'internal locus of control'. They need to reduce medication and
other external pain control factors and improve function.

A group of patients working together provides additional
support and reinforcement for the patient improving long term
prognosis. Pain management programs initially developed to
help return to work and concentrated on spinal pain problems.
However many other chronic pain conditions such as headache,
chronic pelvic pain and irritable bowel syndrome and chronic
medical conditions such as angina benefit from a multidisciplinary approach.

Physical Therapy Approaches

Management techniques used in patients with chronic pain may be subdivided into two major groups. 'Hands-on' methods deal with specific remedial issues. In contrast 'hands-off' methods involve the education and also the use of specific methods which the patients undertake for themselves. For the patient with a chronic condition this latter component can be more effective and avoids the pitfalls of starting a 'hands-on' method for which there is no end point and which may reinforce abnormal coping methods by the patient.

Advice and information

This is a major component of the 'hands-off' methods. The patient needs to know what they can and what they should not do. They need reassurance that physical activity is not harmful and may help in their general wellness. More specific education will be required in for example the patient with back pain who needs to know how to lift and bend, even sit, in ways which will not aggravate their problem. Individualised advice will be required for each patient depending upon their precise complaint.

Exercise and Fitness

A major component in patients with chronic pain is lack of fitness. The patient needs reassurance that they are capable of activity and the need for increased fitness. In addition advice about alternative exercises or methods of exercising which are tailored to individual disabilities.

Sleeping

Specific advice may be required about sleeping posture and the use of, for example, neck support and even bed firmness.

Specific Therapy

There are several methods of stimulation therapy available to the physiotherapist. These include electrical therapy – inferential, short-wave diathermy, and microwave, - ultrasound, and thermal methods using both heat and cold applied to the painful area. These therapies reduce pain by increasing blood flow into the painful area and reduce swelling.

Physical supports/braces

Several methods of bracing or supporting painful areas have been developed. These include such appliances as joint braces, wrist supports, neck collars and spinal braces. Simpler aids such as strapping to support a painful joint are equally effective. These methods help to stabilise and support the joints reducing the degree of pain. Another important area is the system of orthotics allows for better weight transmission through the limb with reduction of other stresses and strains.

Care is needed in selecting appropriate supports and braces, and for the duration of the treatment. Having back pain or neck pain does not need the use of a corset or collar. Used incorrectly appliances may de-function the patient and add to their burden.

Various aids and appliances may be required to for example improve the efficiency of turning a tap, or in the case of grab-bers to save bending or stretching to reach objects thereby min-imising straining and reinjury by the patient.

Manipulation and Massage

Passive and active manipulation of joints or the spine may help by optimising the degree of muscle stretch thereby helping improve contractility and reduction of pain on activity. Advice about stretching prior to exercise and simple massage or manipulations by a spouse or significant other are important.

Manipulative therapy is the basis of osteopathy and chiropractic. These techniques may also involve massage to muscle groups which in turn reduces muscle tight bands and trigger points. Massage is incorporated into osteopathy and aromatherapy.

Functional therapy

It can be important to improve joint and limb function during 'normal' activity. This may require attention to small segments of motor activity in the intended action with concentration on improving these sequentially. In other cases it may be to concentrate on an entire activity but in such a way that the patient is distracted from individual components of the activity. Hydrotherapy, with the use of water for buoyancy and for warmth may ease joint function and range.

Desensitisation

In order to improve function it may be necessary to desensitise a painful area. This can be achieved both directly by increasing contact with the painful area or indirectly by the patient undertaking some activity without realising that they are increasing skin contact with this. These methods are particularly important in some of the conditions in which sensory abnormalities occur, for example in CRPD type 1.

Abbreviations

NSAID	Non-Steroidal Anti-Inflammatory
TENS	Transcutaneous Electrical Nerve Stimulation
SCS	Spinal Cord Stimulator
DREZ	Dorsal Root Entry Zone
NMDA	N-Methyl-D-Aspartamine
CRPD	Complex Regional Pain Disorder
RSD	Reflex Sympathetic Dystrophy
CSF	Cerebrospinal Fluid
o	oral
sc	subcutaneous
im	intramuscular
iv	intravenous
pr	rectal
mg	milligram
μg	microgram
kg	kilogram

Index